KU-546-993

PROSTATE CANCER
Overcoming Denial With Action

A Guide to Screening, Treatment, and Healing

Allen E. Salowe

Afterword by
Michael J. Wehle, M.D.

St. Martin's Griffin ✖ New York

Chapter 1 illustrations courtesy David Bostwick, M.D., Mayo Clinic, Rochester, Minnesota

PROSTATE CANCER: OVERCOMING DENIAL WITH ACTION: A GUIDE TO SCREENING, TREATMENT, AND HEALING. Copyright © 1997 by Quality Medical Publishing, Inc. All rights reserved. Printed in the United States of America. No part of this book may be used or reproduced in any manner whatsoever without written permission except in the case of brief quotations embodied in critical articles or reviews. For information, address St. Martin's Press, 175 Fifth Avenue, New York, N.Y. 10010.

LIBRARY OF CONGRESS CATALOGING-IN-PUBLICATION DATA

Salowe, Allen E.
    Prostate cancer : overcoming denial with action : a guide to screening, treatment, and healing / Allen E. Salowe : afterword by Michael J. Wehle.
        p. cm.
    Includes bibliographical references and index.
    ISBN 0-312-18159-0
    1. Prostate—Cancer—Popular works. I. Title.
RC280.P7S25 1997
616.99'463—dc21
DLC
for Library of Congress   96-50460
                                                       CIP

First published by Quality Medical Publishing, Inc.

First St. Martin's Griffin Quality Medical Publishing Home Health Library Edition: February 1998

10   9   8   7   6   5   4   3   2   1

Acc 331
10 0338178 7

School of N
Derbyshire
London R
DERBY D

Author's Note

This is a story about a personal experience and a profoundly different way of dealing with a health crisis. It describes a single case of prostate cancer and how the forging of a strong patient-physician partnership helped facilitate effective treatment and healing of the disease.

This book's message is not meant to suggest or imply that the courses of treatment chosen by the author and described herein are appropriate for the reader, nor that if they were selected and used, the outcome would be the same. Every effort has been made to ensure the accuracy of the information given here.

Each patient needs to determine his own treatment program through active patient-physician collaboration. Therein lies this story.

University of N
School of N   Midwifery
Derbyshire   Infirmary
London Road
DERBY DE1 2QY

To

Cynthia

Your steadfastness, love, and
caring in the face of untold terror
gave remarkable strength to us both
throughout this experience

♦
_____

Foreword

Everyone agrees that, at present, there is no cure for prostate cancer, except early detection and some chance of removing the cancer entirely through early treatment. Until much more is understood about the disease and more money has been spent to determine not only how to cure it but what causes it, why not use the one procedure that works? *Early detection.*

This is not going to come about unless there is a cessation of the never-ending argument advanced by many professionals, namely, "Until we know screening can be *proved* to improve quality of life, we should not have screening." So the number of men diagnosed with prostate cancer continues to rise yearly, and there are too many naysayers blaming that on better and more frequent detection. Is it more important to satisfy the critics or is the issue saving lives?

Here is the challenge. We have to encourage those men who are in denial about their disease to come forward and help us in our struggle to save them. At the same time, we have to develop proactive efforts to offset the inertia of government regarding prostate cancer and seek positive action. Men must become as organized as the individuals in the breast cancer movement.

Survey Reveals Gap in Patient-Physician Understanding

In the summer of 1995, US TOO! International, Inc., through a grant from Schering/Oncology Biotech, engaged Louis Harris & Associates to interview 1000 of its survivor-members and 200 urologists specializing in prostate cancer. US TOO! promulgates the view that patients should be educated in prostate cancer, should keep good records of treatments and test results, and should take responsibility for decisions regarding their caregivers.

The survey revealed that a high percentage of patients (79%) indicated they had taken an active role in the treatment process. Only 3% did not enter into the decision process.

Despite the fact that all patients interviewed were US TOO! members, there remained a discrepancy between the physician's feelings regarding the exploration of treatment options and the patient's recollection of these discussions.

Since the US TOO! survey was the first of this type ever undertaken, there has been increasing interest generated on the part of survivors, patient organizations, physicians, and professional organizations. Reactions from prominent urologists have been very positive, and there seems to be a good spirit of cooperation in wanting to improve patient-physician relationships and communication.

The goal of the US TOO! organization is to fully educate patients with prostate disease. A man with prostate cancer must be informed about all of his treatment options so that he can work with his physician to decide on the best course of therapy in his particular situation.

The Importance of Screening Tests

Prostate cancer, which strikes about a quarter of a million men annually in the United States alone, is often without recognized symptoms in its early stages. Every 2 minutes a man is diagnosed with prostate cancer, and every 13 minutes a man dies of the disease. In the above-mentioned study, fully two thirds of all prostate cancer patients reported that they had no symptoms before they were diagnosed; physicians estimated that half of their patients on average had symptoms on diagnosis. According to the survey, more than half of all prostate cancer patients are first diagnosed with early-stage (stage A or B, T1 or T2) disease.

"The efforts to educate and screen the growing number of aging men have made an impact," says E. David Crawford, M.D., who was instrumental in founding Prostate Cancer Awareness Week. This annual campaign encourages yearly prostate cancer screening examinations for all men over age 50 and for men over age 40 if they have a family history of the disease.

Discussing Treatment Options With Your Doctor

A clear majority of patients (84%) in the US TOO! survey reported that they had discussed treatment options with their physicians. Although more than 80% of the patients surveyed cited preserving quality of life and delaying disease progression as the main benefits they seek in treatment, physicians consistently thought that survival was the primary concern of their patients. These differences suggest the need for improved communication and collaboration between physicians and patients. While only a minority of patients (8%) were uneasy talking with their doctors, prostate cancer was three times more pronounced in African-American men than in Caucasian men. The disease is particularly aggressive in black men.

"Given the number of options available and the ongoing debate about prostate cancer treatments, patients can seek information not only from their physicians but also social workers, psychologists, and patient advocacy groups who can provide information, education, and support," says Marc B. Garnick, M.D., Associate Clinical Professor of Medicine, Dana-Farber Cancer Institute, a teaching affiliate of the Harvard University Medical School.

Side Effects Are a Patient Concern

Physicians surveyed actually recommended intervention or therapy for only two thirds of their early-stage patients and the less aggressive approach of monitoring the disease or watchful waiting for one third of their patients.

For 45% of the patients surveyed, preserving quality of life is the most important benefit of any treatment. What does this mean? Among prostate cancer patients who face some form of treatment, three key issues stand out: preservation of life, short- or long-term incontinence, and potential impotence. Each patient will place a different priority on the outcome of his treatment, but after preservation of life, there is great concern for quality of life, such as fear of long-term incontinence or impotence.

The US TOO! survey clearly shows greater awareness and activity on the part of prostate cancer patients. But there is much more to be done. Patients must seek information, talk more directly to their doctors, deal with the emotional aspects of their treatments, and take an active role in managing their disease. Their best option is active participation in a support organization such as one of the more than 500 US TOO! prostate cancer support groups.

Henry A. Porterfield

◆

A Physician's Remarks

Most patients have little or no knowledge of the diseases for which they are being treated. Bureaucracy, impersonalization, anxiety about their disease, and questions about their medical care, their physician's expertise, or about available health care facilities often confront and may confound them. To further compound the problem, it is not unusual for more than one approach to treatment of any given illness to exist, with different physicians offering diverse opinions. All these factors unleash a multiplicity of issues that must be considered. Important choices must be made. Indecision and confusion may prove overwhelming to some patients and lead them to abdicate to others the total direction of their care.

As a physician, I have always found that an informed patient is a cooperative patient. All decisions regarding therapy require a careful consideration of risk versus benefit, and it is most important that patients not only understand the various options available, but that they participate in the decision making. Allen Salowe's documentation of his own odyssey through the health care system should help to serve as a road map for any patient also searching for the path to optimal medical care.

The face of medicine is changing. The new health care system tends to encourage volume rather than quality of service. Physicians are not reimbursed for the time spent with a patient nor for the quality of their knowledge. Reimbursements relate to their *doing things* such as tests, procedures, and surgery. Consequently, the tendency may be for many physicians to spend even less time with their patients in explanation and discussion of therapeutic options and the potential side effects of drugs. And because not all physicians are created equal, objective information is very helpful in choosing the appropriate doctor for an individual patient.

The process of medical coaching and collaboration, as outlined by Mr. Salowe with Dr. Lessinger, may assist in this regard as well as directing the education of patients about their disease and prompting them to ask pertinent and meaningful questions of their physician, thereby enabling them to contribute toward taking charge of their own care. This should improve the quality of time patients spend with their physicians and tend to enhance physician-patient relationships.

Mr. Salowe spent many hours educating himself by reviewing the voluminous literature on prostate cancer before he ultimately decided—in conjunction with his physician—on the therapy appropriate for him. I doubt that most patients will have the inclination or commitment to approach such a formidable task. The medical literature on most diseases may even be more extensive, and perhaps more confusing, than that on prostate cancer. More complex organs such as heart, liver, kidney, and brain often present more complicated disease states than the prostate. There can be no substitute for experience, in addition to knowledge, in decision making. Any newly graduated medical student, armed with knowledge but lacking in experience, will readily attest to this.

Patients should be provided with adequate, though not overwhelming, summarized information in a comprehensible format, which will permit them to understand their disease, lead them to ask pertinent, intelligent questions of their physicians, and foster an enhanced interaction regarding therapy. The ultimate risks versus benefits of any treatment presented to the patient can then be weighed in terms of that patient's concerns and in the context of that physician's advice and experience.

Fortunately, it is not necessary for everyone to go to the Mayo Clinic for good care. There are many competent physicians and excellent medical care facilities throughout the country. What the Mayo Clinic did offer to Mr. Salowe was a very personalized and integrated program for patient care. All patients would benefit from similar programs, but at the present time, there is a large vacuum to be filled. Medical coaching, as outlined by Mr. Salowe, is an attempt not only to fill this void, but to enhance such programs.

If medical coaching could be introduced into major medical care facilities, HMOs, and private physicians' offices, it would serve to help create educated patients making informed decisions about their own health, improve the quality of the physician-patient interrelationship, facilitate passage through the tortuous maze of health care bureaucracy, and, most important, help to personalize the medical process.

Harrison A. Fertig, M.D., F.A.C.C.

♦

Preface

The idea for this book surfaced one day when I woke up and realized that I didn't need to call anyone that morning about postoperative care for my prostate cancer surgery—not my urologist, nor his physician's assistant, nor his nurse, nor his secretary. The project, the treatment and healing of what in my case was found to be a locally advanced stage of prostate cancer, had become a full-time management job. After considerable reading and asking a multitude of questions, I had concluded that prostate cancer is a very individualized disease. But that morning I had come to the point at which much of the worst seemed to be behind me.

- I had faced down the terror and uncertainty of prostate cancer.
- I had survived the poking, probing, and cutting.
- I had now healed, for the most part.

In the days following, I gathered together my thoughts and recollections and began to reflect on the countless decisions, the ups and downs. I recalled the anxiousness as well as the feelings of celebration that had been experienced over the previous year.

I felt as though I had been reborn. Nothing looked the same. Nothing sounded the same. Nothing felt the same. Everything now had an aura of beauty surrounding it.

I knew some period of healing still lay ahead of me. So setting about to see these feelings take the form of words, a character at a time, on my word processor seemed cathartic. As the writing project took shape from recall to notes to sentences, it soon proved stimulating, educational, and, I hoped, a service to other men and their families.

I want to acknowledge many for their help. First, Dr. Michael Wehle at the Mayo Clinic Jacksonville, whose review of an early manuscript draft helped improve technical accuracy. His early encouragement and the apparent need to present the patient's point of view became my central mission. Next, several members of the senior staff at Mayo Clinic carefully read the manuscript, which led in turn to Dr. Wehle's contributing the Afterword to this book. My colleague and co-author on another book project, Dr. Leon Lessinger, Eminent Scholar in Education Policy and Economic Development, provided significant support during my healing. He provided the intellectual underpinning for Chapter 8, Medical Coaching and Collaboration, in which the health providers—physician, nurse, physician assistant, technician, and aide—join the patient in viewing collaborative activity as an effective partnership in healing.

A note of thanks to Frank Schnidman, Visiting Professor of Law at the University of Miami, who helped guide me through my earliest introduction to "surfing the Net." Those early Internet days were tedious and awkward, with searches undertaken without the benefit of today's more advanced and powerful search engines. He provided guidance, personal help, and strong cautions. I soon met other prostate cancer patients on-line who, in a good-hearted manner, dispensed first-hand (although sometimes unsubstantiated) advice. Frank is a founder of the American Center for Patient Decision Making, located at *http://www.decision.org* on the Internet.

A special word of thanks goes to Karen Berger, President and Publisher of Quality Medical Publishing. Karen immediately recognized the importance of this book from her personal experience in writing her own book, *A Woman's Decision*, for breast cancer patients, and she agreed to publish my book and direct its distribution to bookstores nationwide. My editor, Suzanne Wakefield, helped focus my writing on those topics that could eventually prove most useful to the broadest audience. From her personal interest, Suzanne urged expansion of Chapter 10, For the Woman Who Cares, and fostered several reference topics that add measurably to the book's practicality.

Finally, warm appreciation to Steven Wilson, Senior Publicist for Borders' Philadelphia bookstore. As an accomplished writer and former book editor, Steve's earliest draft review and insightful suggestions provided me with the necessary guidance to make this a more readable story.

These persons helped make this a more successful writing project. For that they deserve much of the credit for its strength. However, the reader should in no way hold anyone other than the author accountable for any weaknesses in the final product.

Allen E. Salowe

♦

Contents

Chapter 1

Why This Book Was Written

This year more than 300,000 men will receive the devastating news that they have prostate cancer; yet, 8 out of 10 men can't name any of the risk factors of prostate cancer, despite a 90% cure rate if detected early. Although only men have a prostate gland, this event will also affect their wives or partners, family members, co-workers, and friends. The fallout from prostate cancer is not unlike that of a bomb exploding. When it hits, it radiates outward and touches the lives of an astonishing number of people. During this year more than 41,000 men in the United States will die of this dread disease. It has properly been called the *silent killer*, principally because its subtle early warning signals can be all too easily overlooked. More than 1 million persons will be personally affected by prostate cancer each year until much more is learned about its cause and prevention.

I was born in 1933 midway between the stock market crash and the start of World War II. In those years, U.S. birth rates were very low. However, in 1996 the baby boomers (those men born after 1946) began turning 50. Over the next 10 to 15 years, baby boomer men will be entering their earliest years for prostate problems.

The incidence of new prostate cancer cases is almost certain to increase for two distinct reasons. First, prostate cancer screening can be expected to get better as screening technology improves. Second, as mentioned above, the pool of men entering the prime prostate cancer problem years is demographically certain to rise.

Consider a few statistics from the September 1996 Bureau of the Census population estimates. In the United States there are approximately 129 million males. My class—those who have already entered their "prostate trouble" years—includes only 9.2 million men between the ages of 60 and 69. There are 12.2 million men between the ages of 50 and 59—the age range at which the American Cancer Society recommends that prostate screening should begin. In line behind them are hordes of men—19 million, now age 40 to 49, a substantial number of whom can be expected to begin their visits to urologists' offices during the next 10 years for screening examinations. Right behind them another wave is forming—a group of 21 million men, now age 30 to 39, that includes my three sons.

Using current National Cancer Institute probability standards of individuals developing invasive cancer at certain ages, 1 in 6 men over 60 years of age can be expected to be diagnosed with prostate disease. As a result, it is not unreasonable to expect to see twice the number of new prostate cancer cases diagnosed each year using today's technology—and still more as screening technology improves.

Projections of Prostate Cancer Incidence

The American Cancer Society estimates that 317,000 new prostate cancer cases were diagnosed in 1996. In future years we would expect a rise in the total number of new prostate cancer cases found for two reasons. First, we know a great deal about U.S. population projections. Second, we also know statistically when the baby boomers will reach the "prostate trouble" years. Therefore, we applied 1989 to 1993 prostate cancer incidence rates* to U.S. Census Bureau population projections and found that the projected increase in prostate cancer would be as follows:

Between 1996 and 2001	+ 6%
Between 1996 and 2006	+13.8%
Between 1996 and 2010	+23.3%

The 1989 to 1993 incidence rates were multiplied against each age category as it changed annually over time. Although not reflected in these numbers, screening technologies are expected to improve in the future, which may affect the incidence (detection) rate.

In summary, if the incidence rate of prostate cancer remained the same as it is today, the incidence level (new cases found) is certain to increase based on a bulge in the aging male population.

*From Eric J. Feuer, Ph.D., Applied Research Branch, Division of Cancer Prevention and Control, National Cancer Institute, Bethesda, Md.

It simply means that more men and their families need to learn all they can about prostate cancer screening, treatment, and healing.

The clinical incidence of prostate cancer is increasing and has become a matter of concern and study throughout the developed world. "The risk factors for prostate cancer appear to include age, race, positive family history, having undergone a vasectomy, and dietary fat intake," reports Kenneth J. Pienta, M.D., of the Meyer L. Prentis Comprehensive Cancer Center, The Wayne State University School of Medicine, Detroit, Michigan.

It is sometimes difficult to grasp the large numbers associated with "mortality" statistics. Our minds have no framework with which to comprehend a great many deaths. For example, it is one thing to read that more than 41,000 men in the United States will die of prostate cancer in a year; it is quite another when one of those is your loved one. Consider the following data based on American Cancer Society prostate cancer research:

- After age 50, both the incidence of prostate cancer and the rate of death increase exponentially. Prostate cancer incidence increases faster with age than in any other major cancer.
- African-American men have the highest incidence of prostate cancer—reportedly four times greater than that of white males. Veterans Administration (VA) hospital studies conclude that the higher incidence of advanced cases among African-American men may result from negative attitudes toward the health care system and a sense of fatalism about a diagnosis of cancer. African-American men also have a higher incidence of the disease than do black men in Africa or Asia.
- Prostate cancer respects neither education nor socioeconomic class. There seems to be no correlation or sorting of incidence on the basis of socioeconomic factors.
- Prostate cancer is found in 15% to 30% of all men over age 50 and in 60% to 80% of men over age 80. It is not known why some cancers remain dormant while others become clinically detectable.
- Prostate cancer is considered to be genetically linked. The increased risk to sons of fathers who had prostate cancer has been confirmed in European and Japanese studies as well as eight U.S. studies correlating prostate cancer with family history. For

instance, clustering of prostate cancer has been found among Mormon families in Utah; the chances are presently 1 in 2 of a male family member developing prostate cancer, compared with the incidence in the general non-Mormon male population of 1 in 9.

- Sexual behavior, smoking, infectious agents, and occupational hazards seem to have little if anything to do with one's risk of developing prostate cancer. However, a high incidence among farmers has been found. It has been suggested that this may be a result of their frequent contact with chemical fertilizers and pesticides; additional studies are needed.
- Overall, a high intake of dietary fat seems to be associated with a higher risk for developing prostate cancer. "We could virtually destroy prostate cancer by watching what we eat," writes nutritionist Earl Mindel, R.Ph., Ph.D. Similar conclusions have been drawn from studies comparing the incidence of prostate cancer in Japanese men living in Japan compared with that of men of Japanese ancestry living in the United States.

Thus a great many men and their loved ones can expect to travel the same path I did. As one urologist put it, "It's not a question of *whether* you're going to get it, it's *when*." Reportedly, autopsies of men in their nineties show almost universal incidence of the disease.

In my sixty-first year, my annual physical examination was uneventful except for the results from a nonroutine blood test I requested—the prostate-specific antigen (PSA) test—which came back markedly elevated. PSA is a protein marker in the blood that can signal benign as well as malignant prostate disease. Ultimately, my condition was diagnosed as a locally advanced (T3) prostate cancer. At the time I received the news of my sharply elevated PSA, I was not particularly well-informed about prostate cancer; it's fair to say most men are not. As the shock waves of my eventual diagnosis sunk in, I struggled to make sense of the implications for me, my wife, and my family, and I recognized that it was essential to begin an immediate search for more information about the disease and the effect of the available treatment options.

What followed was an often-frustrating health care odyssey during which I experienced, among other things, misdiagnosis and misinformation. I was soon bombarded with confusing, complex, and conflicting medical jargon and, at one point, was led to believe that the best treatment option for me was the one most familiar to whichever doctor I was conferring with at the time. I was to also learn that to a disheartening degree, my experience was not an isolated one.

Three distinct factors prompted my writing this book:

1. I noted during my research that almost every week something shows up in the print media or on television about prostate cancer, but this information is at best abbreviated and at worst misleading. Over the past year or so I have talked with men who have attended a number of prostate cancer support group meetings, yet it has been shockingly apparent to me that too many of these men lack basic knowledge about their prostate gland, and not many more know how to tackle the serious implications of this disease.

2. Physicians' handouts are graphically instructive but are too narrowly focused, antiseptic, and mechanical in tone. Most booklets stress "body part" medicine. At the time of my diagnosis, even the American Cancer Society's booklets seemed badly out of date. A man can quickly become confused by prostate cancer jargon, paralyzed by the uncertain outcomes associated with the array of treatment alternatives, and overly susceptible to outdated physician biases and opinions.

3. The early episodes with my prostate cancer diagnosis and proposed treatment left me distressed. The first doctor misinterpreted my digital rectal examination (DRE), the all-important first-line diagnostic measure for detecting prostate cancer, which I learned is performed with varying degrees of skill. The second doctor downplayed the implications of some of the findings. As one doctor put it, "You go to a surgeon, he sells you surgery; you go to a radiologist, he sells you radiology; you go to a baker, he sells you bread." I needed to find and understand up-to-date medical information, not merely accept routine or dismissive answers.

First Step: The Learning Process

These and other events quickly convinced me that I had better take an active role in managing my own case (whatever that was to come to mean). I decided to look on the diagnosis, treatment, and healing of my suddenly discovered case of prostate cancer as I would a professional project and to find a way to become part of a strong patient-physician team effort.

Thus far I am a survivor. That means that I am *healed, not cured.* Although the major signals flash all clear, my life has changed forever. With cancer, a person senses that he or she is never quite out of the woods. During the period of time described in this book, I underwent more than a technical learning experience about a disease; it was an *educative experience* as well—a profound shift in my view of the world—as I came face-to-face with the realization of my own mortality.

During this learning process I digested a great deal of information about survival and overseeing one's health. Having been transformed in a single moment from a seemingly healthy guy to a prostate cancer patient, it was apparent that the adjustment would mean more than grasping a set of facts about the physiology of this disease and its treatment alternatives. It gradually sank in that I had embarked on a new life experience, during which I had to constantly search for the meaning in each step of the healing process.

As I traveled farther into the long, dark tunnel of intensive health care, it also became quite clear that this was not going to be a pleasure trip. Through the haze of the early period following this diagnosis, I began to realize that facing major surgery for a life-threatening disease, with the prospect of permanent side effects, is light-years from any previous life experience.

Each time I donned a hospital gown that never quite covered everything and submitted my body parts to the health care professionals, I felt more vulnerable. It was as though I was surrendering all power and control over my life with each event. Little did I realize that "power and control" would also come to include those essential bodily functions I had taken so much for granted—one since abandoning diapers and the other since puberty. Every episode drove home the idea that to survive this encounter intact and to heal effectively required my playing an active role in all treatment decisions.

This book is not meant to be a dry recitation of medical facts and events, nor a presentation of a universally effective treatment regimen. It is the story of my personal experiences. It is the private story about one man's encounter with a locally advanced stage of prostate cancer—fortunately, not the most advanced stage, but too darn close for comfort. I hope to share insights that may lead you to determine how best to take charge of your own health care.

There are several good technical guides for those who are dealing with prostate cancer, among which I recommend *The Prostate: A Guide for Men and the Women Who Love Them* by Dr. Patrick Walsh and Janet Farrar Worthington. Walsh and Worthington have written a detailed and sympathetic book. One concern is that the book may inadvertently focus the man's attention on *retaining* his potency postsurgically rather than keeping his eye on the target of *overcoming* this disease. Nonetheless, the book is a valuable resource. *Prostate Cancer: A Family Guide to Diagnosis, Treatment and Survival* by Dr. Sheldon Marks is a detailed book written in the question and answer format. It is an effective discussion for patients and their families who want to understand the multiple dilemmas and management issues associated with prostate cancer. Marks' book and the Walsh-Worthington book are about 300 pages each, and absorbing so much information could prove an overwhelming task for a newly diagnosed patient or his family, who are faced with the fast-moving and changing events confronting them in the critical first days and weeks following initial diagnosis. *How I Survived Prostate Cancer . . . and So Can You* by James Lewis, Jr., Ph.D., is a technical handbook written for patients by a survivor. In lucid language it presents many aspects of coping with prostate cancer. *My Prostate and Me: Dealing with Prostate Cancer* by William Martin, Ph.D.—who reportedly survived his cancer treatment with very few side effects—conveys basic medical information about the disease and treatment in a straightforward, nontechnical book that can be read in an evening. A valuable recent addition to the library of books on the subject is *Prostate Cancer: What Every Man—and His Family—Needs to Know* by David G. Bostwick, M.D., et al., written for the American Cancer Society. The text is a thorough treatment of the subject and is quite readable.

I have written this book in the hope that one more prostate cancer patient and his family may benefit from my experiences and be motivated to set aside denial about his situation and take charge of and responsibility for his case; that one more physician or other member of the health provider team might choose to encourage a collaborative patient-physician team effort; and that one more family might be spared the anguish of an untimely loss.

Understanding the Basics: Being Evaluated for Prostate Disease

Only men have a prostate gland. It is located deep in the lower abdomen just below the bladder and behind the penis (Figure 1). Its purpose is to generate prostatic fluid, which becomes part of the man's semen—the milky fluid ejaculated during male orgasm. Running through the middle of the prostate is the urethra, the tube carrying urine from the bladder through the penis (Figure 2). Thus the prostate is part of both the urinary and reproductive systems (Figure 3). The prostate is surrounded by a membrane or *capsule* and has several distinct *zones* (Figures 4 and 5).

In a young boy, the prostate gland is about the size of an almond. At puberty the prostate gland begins to grow as it readies itself to perform its role in the male reproductive process. Its dimensions level off to about the size of a walnut shortly thereafter. As a man moves into his forties, the prostate begins to grow again, fueled by the body's testosterone levels and other factors. A man's prostate gland may continue to grow well into his seventies and eighties. My father had

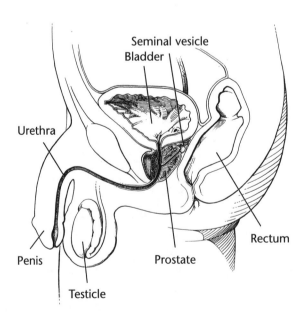

Figure 1   Male anatomy, showing the location of the prostate.

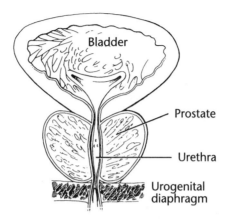

Figure 2   The prostate, indicating the position of the urethra.

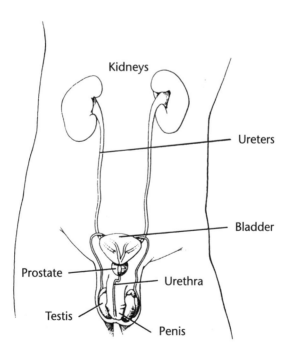

Figure 3   The male urinary system.

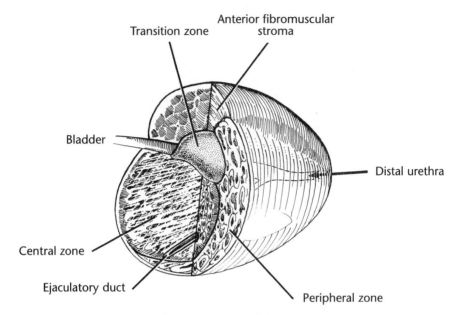

Figure 4   Zones of the prostate.

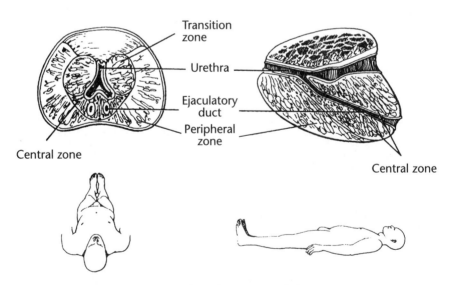

Figure 5   Side and top views of the prostate.

surgery in his early eighties for benign prostatic hyperplasia, a condition characterized by an enlarged prostate without cancer.

Because of its strategic location, the prostate plays an important role in urination. Sound preventive care for the prostate starts with a DRE administered by a competent urologist. Former GIs will remember this part of the trip down the line.

Following some reassuring words such as "Let's have a look," the doctor slips on a rubber glove, covers his index finger with K-Y lubricant, and inserts the finger into the patient's rectum, probing to determine the "feel" of the prostate. The doctor evaluates the size and hardness of the prostate and explores for any suspicious lumpiness that may signal an abnormality. This procedure is quick, painless, and essential, and it is over in a matter of seconds.

Abnormalities in prostate size can eventually cause urinary blockage. A firmness or unusual hardening—a nodule—may be an early sign of prostate cancer. In its earliest stages, cancerous prostate cells may have been growing for 10 years before their accumulation reaches the size that can be felt by the urologist's well-trained finger (a nodule of about 1 cm, or the size of a small sugar cube), a good example of the value of early detection. After age 40 it is advisable for a man to make DRE prostate screening an annual event.

The value of the PSA test for cancer screening remains controversial. Blood is drawn and sent to the laboratory for testing. PSA is a protein molecule produced almost exclusively by the prostate and found at a low level in the blood. When a problem starts to arise in the prostate, the increased concentrations of PSA leak into the bloodstream. A rising PSA level can signal infections, benign prostatic hyperplasia, or cancer. It is significant to note that the PSA test is not a routine part of a standard battery of blood tests. I learned this lesson the hard way.

An initial prostate screening evaluation includes both the DRE and PSA test. In men over 50 years of age, the American Cancer Society recommends both tests annually. For men with a family history of prostate cancer and African-American men, age 40 is the recommended starting point for annual prostate screening examinations.

If either a PSA score is out of bounds or the DRE yields a suspicious feel (both reliable indicators of the presence of cancer), it is usually suggested that the patient undergo transrectal ultrasonography so the urologist can "map" the prostate gland. At the same time, if warranted, the urologist may perform a biopsy, that is, anesthetize the patient in the operating room and snip small amounts of tissue from the prostate for more detailed analysis by the pathology laboratory. These bits of tissue yield samples of cancerous cellular structure, allowing the physician to grade and score the patient's prostate cancer.

If the results of ultrasound and the biopsy confirm the presence of prostate cancer, the attending urologist may decide (although not in all cases) to order two additional noninvasive tests to determine whether there has been any discernible spread of cancer to any other sites in the body—a bone scan and a computed tomography (CT) scan. Both tests are painless and can best be imagined as advanced forms of an x-ray evaluation.

The primary purpose of the bone scan is to determine whether any cancer can be detected as having spread to the bones. A radioactive dye is injected into the bloodstream and is absorbed by the bones, which allows the bones to show up more clearly on film. The dye is later excreted in the urine.

The CT scan produces a series of x-ray films. The patient lies comfortably on a table and is slowly moved into a tunnel while a space-age machine rotates all of the way around the body. A computer translates information about the body into cross-sectional views. Occasionally this procedure is used to determine whether any cancer has spread to the adjacent lymph nodes, although the lymph node dissection described later is a more direct (although invasive) approach.

Prostate Cancer Grading and Staging

Urologists use a standard scoring system to rank the seriousness of a patient's prostate cancer case. Under the Gleason method (see Chapter 4 and Appendix C), which uses a scale of 1 to 10, my prostate cancer disease was scored Gleason 9. In Gleason terms, a lower number is much more favorable. A cancer graded Gleason 10 has spread to other parts of the body and is beyond cure. Among other factors, a Gleason score identifies the aggressiveness of the cancer. When examined microscopically, the cells of my prostatic tissue were found to be *poorly differentiated,* which describes a bizarre-shaped, rapidly growing cell pattern.

Prostate cancers are also *staged.* In the older (Whitmore-Jewett) staging system, which uses A to D, the "school report card" standard is still much favored. Mine was a stage C cancer, defined as cancer cells that have spread outside the prostate capsule and perhaps to the lymph node tissues near the prostate. Under the newer staging system, this cancer would be classified as T3 (see Appendix C). I also overheard my case being called a "Big C" prostate cancer. At that moment, I felt as though a time bomb were ticking inside my body.

Over the past 3 years, since starting down the road to prostate cancer survival, I have been especially troubled that few prostate cancer patients with whom I spoke knew these and other basic facts about their own cases. It is not at all clear whether their doctors did not effectively explain the findings and their implications, or whether these men, as is true of many patients, preferred not to know or remember important details. Also interestingly, although not all that surprising, most wives with whom I spoke seemed to be better informed about their husband's condition than he was.

One urologist-surgeon shared the distressing finding that among his Latino patients, there was a high incidence of denial after the man received the news about his prostate cancer. In fact, a patient seldom returned on his own for follow-up treatment. It is never easy for man to face a direct and serious threat to his sexual potency. We hear the term *macho* frequently, but many people may not realize that the Spanish word from which it is derived, *machismo*, denotes an exaggerated sense of masculine pride, a societal belief that it is unmanly to concede any weakness, including disease.

When a person receives a diagnosis of cancer, he or she is immediately confronted with a series of new challenges. First, there is shock, anxiety, and uncertainty. Gradually, questions begin to surface. Too often, the patient or family member is too timid to pursue these concerns, but that is exactly what needs to be done. We may not immediately know the right questions to ask. Sometimes we know the questions we would like to ask, but the physician or health care professional seems reluctant or too impatient to sit still and give straight answers. Early on in my case, my wife asked the important questions while I listened and sensed my world swirling with change, moment by moment.

The farther I ventured into the surreal landscape of prostate cancer, the more apparent it seemed to me that *each case is a statistical case of one.* Not all cancer cases are created alike. There are enough distinct characteristics that each patient needs to learn the implications of his particular diagnosis, the most reasonable treatment options, and what the process of healing is likely to be in his particular case.

No one can take better care of you than you! This is a story about taking control of your own case of prostate cancer. It is about managing your predicament as one would oversee an important project, becoming involved—no, immersed—in grasping the implications of diagnostic information, comprehending the benefits and risks of alternative treatments, and preparing yourself for what lies ahead during the healing process. It is about the search for meaning in the face of pain and the temporary or permanent loss of control over part of your body. Finally, it is also about sharing the celebrative experiences—those events that periodically come about as the result of overcoming seemingly insurmountable odds.

A well-worn Chinese proverb reminds us that a trip of a thousand miles must begin with a single step. In healing prostate cancer, a life-threatening disease, the journey must begin with *the right mind-set*. A full and open dialogue between patient and physician is vital to arriving at an accurate diagnosis and a positive patient attitude, both of which are absolutely essential to effective treatment strategy.

Norman Cousins, acclaimed journalist and editor of the *Saturday Review,* was the author of some 20 books, including *Anatomy of an Illness,* in which he described his own healing through the use of laughter to achieve a disease-defeating mind-set. In his book, *Head First,* Cousins wrote: "In our medical economy dominated by third-party payors—insurance companies, the government, health plans, etc.—the harsh reality is that doctors get paid mostly for tests and procedures. Even more serious is the reduced time available for careful questioning by the physician. Technology can supply measurements, but only the patient can supply essential background information."

Men—The Fixers and Doers

Faced with these new realities, the mission of managing my own interests gradually began to take shape. My image of myself was of a person in command of himself, capable and sure in most situations. Suddenly I was confronted with an overwhelming awareness that something was happening in my body over which I had no control. I couldn't simply "fix" this thing.

Some men are fix-up specialists; they can plan repairs and handle a multitude of improvements around the house. Others are weekend sportsmen, with the requisite skills and apparatus of the game. (In golf, a sport I gave up 20 years ago, I found that the apparatus was more often apparent than the skills.) Men who are athletic and involved in a very physical sport may think they are invulnerable. Some men hold the belief that nothing bad or permanent can happen to them—they think they are bulletproof; they never dwell on how fragile life really is.

Many men, whatever their background, find that they already have strong project management skills, whether these have been gained from running a product campaign, planning and executing a major remodeling project on the house, or coordinating a family trip. Project management of one's own health is a matter of applying these same skills to an event of enormous significance—the treatment and healing of a life-threatening disease.

In *Real Moments,* Barbara DeAngelis, Ph.D., wrote: "Men have been trained since the beginning of time to be good at doing—they hunted, they built, they protected. That was their role, and thus it was through their work, their toil, and their accomplishment that they defined themselves, and found their value."

A choice between the present and the future is one of the hardest decisions you could ever make. Will you decide on a course of treatment that has the potential for causing short- or long-term side effects, or will you elect to do nothing at all and face the consequences? The decision influences whether you will stay the course or quit—whether you will hold out against the odds or be ensnared by circumstances. Do you settle with the first opinion or challenge the initial findings, even if it makes matters more complicated? How much uncertainty about future outcomes—unpleasant side effects—can a man live with? Is it better to accept prostate cancer and shrug, "That's life," or to search for new meaning in each remaining day? Should you yield all control and decision making to others, or take charge yourself?

In my case, values instilled in childhood as well as my schooling and work experiences over many years helped to prepare me to think and act as a project planner and manager—a decision maker. Since I had no apparent physical symptoms before my diagnosis of prostate cancer, I immediately felt personally challenged by the situation. Later, on reflection, I realized that my body had been sending me "smoke signals" for about 2 years—increased urinary frequency and urgency, and slight discomfort—which I mistakenly attributed to just getting a little older. I had not recognized any of the common warning signs (and more subtle hints) associated with prostate disease. Like most men, I was just too busy; I was doing my thing. I was not listening with an "inner ear"; I didn't know enough to pay attention to what my body was trying to tell me.

Initially, I thought that there must have been a mistake in the blood test results. My family doctor's physical examination and the blood test results from the laboratory did not match up. The doctor said I was fine; my PSA level said otherwise. And I felt fine—nothing obvious hurt or felt wrong.

As you learn more about the *serious* warning signs of prostate cancer, you discover that if you fail to heed the signals until you actually begin to feel the "real and painful" symptoms of this disease, the cancer will most likely have spread to other parts of the body. At that point, if is often too late for the cancer to be surgically removed and thus completely cured.

I knew my family history well; I was a prime candidate for this disease. So despite my initial reaction of denial and disbelief, I was not too surprised when I got the news. Frankly, once I was given the word that it was cancer, I was "hell bent" to go after the damn thing. Early on, my wife remarked about my rather matter-of-fact take-charge attitude toward the news and initiating the first steps toward a cure. This did not mean that I lacked strong feelings and emotions about the turn of events. Rather, this threat focused my attention on getting results now and on the future—on things yet to be fulfilled in a life not yet ready to be closed. Taking charge also helped me to reduce the focus on what could easily have become a cycle of self-absorption.

I needed to deal with events as they unfolded. It was essential to gather the tools of knowledge, find allies and resources in the medical profession, and focus my energies on the kind of problem solving I already knew I could do. What followed was a process of managing my own project—a healing process that is managed to this day in close partnership with my urologist and his staff.

Noted Dr. DeAngelis: "Men are at home in the physical world, the world of the concrete. They feel comfortable with what they can see and touch and measure. They are goal oriented. That is why they put such a high value on doing, because it provides a result that fits into their model of what is worthwhile."

This is also a story within a story. At one level I have related my experience in taking charge of my own prostate cancer case, the interaction with health care professionals at every critical step along the path from diagnosis to healing. At another level, this story is a guide to jointly managing a serious health crisis—whatever the disease—among patients, their families, and their physicians.

The concept of *medical coaching and collaborative medicine* will be introduced in Chapter 8 for serious consideration by health care professionals as well as for use by the informed patient. Medical coaching or medical collaboration is a process whereby the effective involvement of the patient in his or her own health maintenance and treatment is advanced by the physician to strengthen the patient's healing. At the same time, it augments the caregiver's effectiveness and efficiency through the forging of a working patient-physician team. Medical coaching can help attain significant and cost-effective results in the face of the continuous economic pressures and changing health care standards.

Chapter 2

Preparing to Take Charge

The Task of Project Management

When I was a child, our family doctor always seemed to be at our house. He was, as I recall, a kind and gentle man. He would sit on the side of my bed with a stethoscope around his neck, like someone straight out of a Norman Rockwell poster.

As far back as I can remember, I was recuperating from something: broken bones, pneumonia, or gashes requiring sutures. When I was 3 years old, my older brother Bill, age 16 and probably 160 pounds, thought I looked so cute dancing in front of a mirror that he tackled me and broke my leg. (That may be one reason I have never been crazy about dancing.) My sister Shirley, 8 years older than I was, gave me most of my scars, usually in response to my taunting her. I spit, she chased. I went right through a glass door. Only my sister Beattie, 16 years my senior, had not tried to destroy me. At the end of World War II, penicillin, the new wonder drug, rescued me from mustard plaster treatments and helped me to beat off the last of three childhood bouts with pneumonia.

Despite the best efforts of my older siblings, I survived to grow up, imbued with an understanding of the importance of education and having some sense of purpose. My folks had come to this country separately from the Ukraine before World War I, met one another here in America, married, and had four children.

My mother first lived on New York's Lower East Side, worked in a shirt factory, but never learned to read or write. Yet she saw to it that her two girls and two boys all went to college. She taught us the value of "learning a living." And a family gathering was never over until we each told her what we had planned for the next day and for the rest of the week.

My father, with his five brothers and two sisters, beat it out of the old country before all of the boys were conscripted into the Czar's army. In New Jersey he built a small dry cleaning business with a top-notch reputation for quality and service. Dad taught me early and often what it meant to care for the customer's needs. One day he took me to task for parking my new (10-year-old used) car in front of his store, forcefully reminding me, "That is where the customers park." Looking back, it is easy to see that my parents instilled in me attitudes they valued highly and that these attitudes influenced my career. It is also clear that my early experiences helped shape my actions after my diagnosis of prostate cancer.

Just after college my first job, as a medical detail person for an ethical (prescription-only) drug company, was to present new pharmaceutical products to doctors and hospitals. Through that experience I learned a great deal about the minute-by-minute pressures under which physicians, nurses, and other health care workers must function. Although this was quite a few years ago, the volume of information then being circulated in the health care field was enormous. Several years later I consulted to a number of pharmaceutical companies on methods for streamlining the detailing and delivery of medical information. To this day it remains a daunting task for doctors to keep pace with new studies, new drugs, and new protocols. I truly admire their dedication.

Over the past 40 years I have run a number of important projects for companies. Those assignments gave me important experiences, among which were lessons learned in how to organize and manage teams. My responsibilities also included collecting, assimilating, and synthesizing large amounts of conflicting information. My projects frequently called for conferring with or directing persons with considerably greater specialized knowledge than my own. It also meant coordinating the efforts of people from different levels of an organization and at times being called on to make hard decisions or sometimes to pursue a course that was controversial.

Over the same period I raised two families. The first 20 years I helped my first wife, Suzi, raise our three sons—Marshall, Kenneth, and Warren. Each had highly individual needs. Anyone who has raised a family knows that children are a major project to manage! We lived in New Jersey, Dallas, Memphis, and Charlotte. Most of those young family years involved formative parenting. The teen years were a struggle with differences in values and lifestyles between our generations and the early adult years focused on their getting their formal education. Suzi and I then divorced, and I began the project of starting over in a new phase of my life.

When I met my present wife, Cynthia, she too was starting over, a widow with two children, Erica and Bill. We married and currently live and work in Florida. Our five children, all in their thirty-something years, have grown into fine adults. All finished college and all have built healthy personal and professional lives. We also have four grandchildren, Billy, Jr., Geoffrey, Rachel, and Alex.

Unfortunately, each of my three sons has a three-times-greater likelihood of developing prostate disease than the average man. Prostate cancer is now acknowledged to be a genetically transmitted disease. My older brother had prostate cancer, and he is a survivor. Two first cousins died of the disease. Regardless of professional debate on the merits of early prostate screening, I have alerted each of my sons to begin his prostate screening testing not later than his fortieth birthday.

Looking Past the Headlines

Remember when butter was bad and margarine was good? These days, butter is better and margarine is not so good. Oat bran is another example. When a study showed that it helped lower cholesterol levels, manufacturers of oatmeal and other oat-based products could not keep up with demand. Another study then showed that oat bran did not lower cholesterol. Demand for oat bran plummeted. Later, a third study confirmed the earlier report that oat bran helped. Now we have oat bran bagels, breads, and cereals on the breakfast table. Those two examples exemplify the confusing information we receive about what is healthful and what is not. What is a health-conscious person to do with conflicting information about what is appropriate for maintaining our well-being?

It is easy to get mired in the differences between *screening* for prostate cancer and *early detection* of the disease. According to Dr. Otis

Brawley, senior investigator in the division of Cancer Prevention and Control at the National Cancer Institute, "Screening can be bad because in some men prostate cancer grows so slowly that they are likely to die of other causes before the cancer becomes serious." Brawley notes that "the side effects of surgery—including incontinence and impotence—may be worse than the cancer, since the cancer would otherwise never alter their lifestyle."

The U.S. Preventive Health Services Task Force issued updated guidelines in 1995 that may be used for insurance purposes. In its report it made the following recommendations against screening for prostate cancer: "*Routine screening for prostate cancer with digital rectal examinations, serum tumor markers (e.g., prostate-specific antigen), or transrectal ultrasound is not recommended.*"

An informed consent form used by Kaiser Permanente (Colorado) medical offices for men who have no signs, symptoms, or history of prostate cancer provides a quandary for the patient as he prepares to sign it. In part, it reads (emphasis in original):

There is no proof that early detection of prostate cancer with PSA screening will be effective in improving your chances of survival. By consenting to a PSA test, you believe that the potential benefits of diagnosing asymptomatic prostate cancer may outweigh the risks of the tests and treatments. By choosing *not* to have a PSA test, you believe that the potential risk of tests and treatments may outweigh the benefits of diagnosing asymptomatic prostate cancer.

The *Journal of the National Cancer Institute* confronts the controversy in this way: "Researchers and clinicians agree that screening, early detection, and treatment are the central belief of cancer control—but, as yet, unproved when dealing with prostate cancer." The Canadian Task Force on the Periodic Health Examination concluded (emphasis added): "Since there is *no alternative technology* that performs better than the DRE in detecting early-stage prostate cancer and since the burden of the illness is potentially heavy, DRE should not be excluded from periodic health examination of asymptomatic men over 40 years of age."

The American Cancer Society and the American Urological Association both agree that regular screening for prostate cancer is in the patient's best interest at the recommended age levels. What a man needs to confront head-on are equivocal recommendations at best and the potential for deadly results at worst. Ultimately, the decision whether you should have regular tests for prostate cancer—and what those tests should be—is a matter for you and your physician to decide together.

The debate rages internationally—in Australia, the PSA test is not widely recommended. However, there is an Australian Prostate Cancer Society with a home page on the World Wide Web. Although the French have long doubted the benefits of widespread PSA testing, the death of former French President François Mitterand after a long battle with prostate cancer emphasized the importance of screening. Recently, Thailand's Minister of Labor succumbed to prostate cancer. The *Malaysian Doctor,* a professional journal, reported on early-stage prostate studies in the United Kingdom. In 1996, the First International Consultation of Prostate Cancer was organized by the World Health Organization (WHO) and International Union Against Cancer. In its preconference announcement, organizers noted the following (emphasis in original):

At a time when clinical decisions are becoming *highly standardized* in most areas of medicine, they are still *complex* and *confusing* in many areas of prostate cancer management, primarily because of two factors:
1. The number and variety of *treatment options* and their possible combinations (given concurrently or sequentially) are *increasing rapidly.*
2. The *benefit* of one treatment over another (or sometimes watchful waiting) *has not been precisely determined* by randomized prospective trials.
Recent practice surveys have shown that the *management of this disease* (by basic scientific standards) is *unacceptably disparate,* leaving some patients undertreated or overtreated. The *negative impact* of this situation of the *quality* and *cost effectiveness* of care is obvious.

My first urologist told me that had a man 45 years of age developed an aggressive prostate cancer such as mine, he would have been dead in a year. Not all prostate cancer cases are created equal. My second urologist assured me that if my case had gone undetected and untreated, I would most assuredly have suffered a painful death in a year.

If prostate cancer is reportedly so slow growing, why do some cases progress so rapidly? Tumors, any tumors, that are found to be malignant are life threatening! In prostate cancer they fit three classifications:

1. Localized tumors that remain within the wall of the prostate capsule where they began;
2. Regional tumors that invade neighboring tissues such as other parts of the urogenital system; and
3. Metastasized tumors, which are cells that break away from the primary tumor and have spread to other parts of the body—most commonly, bones, liver, and lungs.

Different cancers grow at different rates of speed. In discussing cancer growth the doctor often refers to the doubling rate—the time it takes for the total number of cells to increase by 100%. A noncancer example may help illustrate the awesome threat from the doubling rate of cancer growth:

Lily pads grow on a lake. The number of lily pads doubles every day. It will take 30 days for the lily pads to cover the entire surface of the lake. How much of the lake is covered with lily pads on the twenty-ninth day? Answer: one half of the lake is covered. With doubling, there is as much growth on the thirtieth day as took place in the first twenty-nine days.

Reportedly, most prostate cancers are slow growing, with doubling rates measured in years. However, there are three factors that alter the slow growth rule. First, the larger the tumor, the more likely it is to grow rapidly to adjacent tissues. Second, the more orderly the cell formation (well differentiated), which means the bad cells resemble the good cells, the less likely the spread of the cancer. On the other hand, 15% of prostate cancer cases reportedly consist of poorly differentiated cells and these are more likely to accelerate spreading, as with the lily pads on the lake. Third, the density of tumor invasiveness of small blood vessels signals another potential for rapid growth—the higher the density, the more likely the cancer cells are to grow and spread (metastasize).

Based on traditional practices, men are often told that prostate screening is not necessary until age 50 or 60 unless symptoms arise.

Based purely on statistical occurrence, many doctors and most press reports characterize prostate cancer as a typically slow-growing disease in about 85% of cases.

Although the disease is less likely to be found in younger men (under age 40) the life expectancy of a man in his seventies may still exceed 10 years or more. Widely reported in the news is the fact that prostate cancer patients over 70 years of age are often told that something else will probably kill them before prostate cancer gets them. Therefore, doing nothing (watchful waiting is the clinical term) is thought to be the best course of treatment for most older patients. That may prove to be true—but only if the cancer is first found and then determined to have the essential characteristics that lead the patient and physician to conclude it is probably slow growing.

Recently, a 71-year-old prostate cancer patient called to discuss my experiences with a specific course of treatment. He had been diagnosed with a fast-growing prostate tumor, yet his actuarial life expectancy still exceeded the "death countdown" from his prostate cancer. Should he have just followed the standard recommendations of the experts? The press reports?

One of the unacceptable realities of the widespread debate about prostate cancer PSA screening comes down to age and money. In many respects this issue mirrors the growing debate about the increasing number of elderly and whether Social Security and Medicare can pay for all of the needed care. First, it is a given that prostate cancer incidence rises as the population grows older. Second, recognizing the growth of the aging U.S. male population, there is widespread concern among health care plans and insurance companies about the potential cost of treating the large numbers of prostate cancer cases that would most likely result from widespread PSA screening. In short, who wants to pay for treating so many older men who are eventually going to die of something anyway?

It is important to watch out for medical absolutes, especially those that may be summarized in a newspaper article or television news show or even imparted by well-meaning friends or prostate cancer support group members. You must gather together a broad array of facts to protect yourself.

The diagnosis of prostate cancer does not mean death. Early detection is still the best way to get a jump on any cancer while it is still in its earliest stages. If you are over 40 years of age, an annual prostate screening is a very good idea. For the majority of men, such a step will mean finding out that you do not have cancer. And the peace of mind will be worth it. For the relatively small percentage of men screened who do in fact find that they have cancer, the benefits are even greater. As with most cancers, the earlier it is detected in the prostate the more options there are for treatment and the greater the potential survival time.

Much of the debate surrounding prostate cancer screening does not relate to whether screening detects cancer earlier. It centers on whether treatment is necessary. There is no question that prostate cancer is detected earlier through screening. The question ultimately comes down to this: What do you do once the disease is diagnosed? My best advice: *Have a DRE performed by a skilled urologist and* check *your PSA level regularly.* Detect prostate disease early to save your life; 25% of men diagnosed die of this disease—the same death rate as with breast cancer in women.

Are You Prepared to Take Charge?

The French scientist Poincare is credited with having been the first to say, "Discovery favors the prepared mind." Similarly, Louis Pasteur stated, "In the field of observation, chance favors the prepared mind," after relating how he came upon the purification method that now bears his name. Still others credit the words to mathematician Blaise Pascal. Studies have shown that a DRE alone would miss a third of prostate cancers. Ultrasonography would also have missed a third of cancers. The PSA test has the lowest error rate of all tests.

The combination of a urologist-administered DRE *and* a PSA test is a check and balance. In my situation, the family doctor missed feeling the tumor when he performed a DRE. Fortunately, the PSA blood test, so readily dismissed by government study teams, raised the red flag. As an example of the reverse, both the commander of Operation Desert Storm, General Norman Schwarzkopf, and NFL Hall of Fame member Len Dawson saw their PSA blood test results come back *within normal range.* But through DREs performed by *skilled* urologists, the suspicious areas were discovered.

Everyday events and ordinary skills can help prepare you for grappling with a life-threatening project assignment. Something as simple as home gardening can serve as a mental model for managing a project. The garden must be planned, cultivated, planted, cared for, and protected from insect infestation. It is an ongoing process. So too is personal health management.

Forging the Patient-Physician Partnership in the Age of Managed Care

In an age in which health maintenance organizations (HMOs) and managed care systems have rapidly replaced the once intimate relationship between patient and personal physician, it is all the more critical that patients learn to take better care of themselves, both physically and spiritually. In this sense I am speaking of the personal responsibility, both physically and mentally, that the patient must now take on to help ensure his or her personal well-being. We cannot afford to be passive passengers; we must be copilots of our own health care decisions.

The take-charge patient may at first be resisted, or worse yet, even be resented at times by health care professionals. On the other hand, the best physicians encourage a high degree of patient involvement, although the physician cannot allow you to practice medicine without a license. Your care must be viewed as a collaborative and cooperative effort.

It is important to recognize that many factors influence the way you and your doctor view medical care. Medicine does not provide a monitor screen with black and white answers; the practice of medicine is an art as well as a science, and patient and physician must accept that there are many shades of gray. Medicine is a here-and-now, at-this-moment proposition. Looking backward is useful only as a diagnostic aid. It is a waste of precious energy to think about what might have been.

It is almost impossible to identify the "best" doctors in a particular specialty. Most people will obtain all or most of their medical care near where they live. Thus it is important to identify doctors who are among the best in your own community. There are doctors who, on paper at least, meet every professional standard but who are simply not good doctors. There are also doctors who are outstanding leaders in their fields because of professional activities but who are not particularly effective or perhaps even active in patient care. The chief criterion by which patients select doctors is *reputation.*

Most doctors are on the medical staff of one or more hospitals. If a doctor does not have admitting privileges or is not on the attending staff of a hospital, you may want to consider selecting another doctor. It can be very difficult to determine whether the lack of hospital appointment is for good reason or not.

The one type of experience that should specifically be queried is the doctor's track record with a particular procedure, especially a surgical one. You should not hesitate to ask how many times the doctor has performed a procedure and with what degree of success. Practice may not lead to perfection, but it improves skills and enhances the probability of success.

Managing your own health care focuses your attention on personal strengths rather than on weaknesses. This is useful in relieving the feelings of helplessness and depression that may arise during serious illness. It concentrates on taking the beautiful, robust mechanism that is the body, couples it with a positive take-charge mindset, and forges a linkage with members of the health care team. It is the win-win approach that served me well in the events I will be describing.

Accountability Is Your Bottom Line

Members of an HMO program or any other kind of managed health care plan face some special circumstances. First, in managed health care plans, the doctors, nurses, and other health care providers are "prepaid"; this is different from traditional insurance plans that pay out for treatment the patient gets when they are sick. For a small copayment or fee, an HMO typically provides screening physical examinations, checkups, and diagnostic procedures, as well as the medical or surgical care you might need. These are often referred to as "wellness programs," which are designed to keep the patient from becoming sick, which in turn saves the patient money in the long run. Patients covered by Medicare are being encouraged to join HMOs to supplement their coverage.

There are several different kinds of HMOs. If the patient is a member of a managed care organization (MCO)—of which an HMO is a form—it is particularly important to determine and fully understand the terms and conditions that govern particular circumstances. A staff model HMO employs its doctors on salary; a group HMO comprises several physician group practices that have contracted with one another to work together to provide services. In independent practice associations (IPAs), the HMO contracts with individual doctors or physician groups to serve HMO patients, in addition to their non-HMO patients. There are mixed-model plans that combine some variation of these types. In a point of service (POS) HMO, the patient is allowed to go outside the HMO network of doctors to look for specialist care, at some increase in cost.

Managed care programs in the form of HMOs evolved in the mid-1970s as prepaid programs featuring preventive care coverage. Notwithstanding the variations in possible plans, the bottom line means accountability to the patient and the purchaser of those services. And since this is your life and health, the same principles of patient-driven initiatives, as described throughout this book, still apply.

- Talk to your employer/sponsor or program administrator.
- Review your findings and discuss your options for screening or treatment.
- Consider your need to go outside the system for help.
- Whatever you decide, put your life and health first.

Information Is at the Heart of Managed Care

In June 1994, the National Committee for Quality Assurance (NCQA) began regular and full disclosure to the public of health plans' accreditation status. The Accreditation Status List, updated on the fifteenth of each month, catalogs all plans that have an accreditation status with NCQA, all plans with pending accreditation decisions, and all plans scheduled for review. An independent nonprofit organization, NCQA is widely recognized as the leader in the effort to assess, measure, and report on the quality of health care provided by the nation's MCOs. About half the nation's HMOs have been reviewed as part of the NCQA accreditation process.

NCQA is a nationally recognized evaluation that health care purchasers, regulators, and consumers can use to assess MCOs, such as HMOs. NCQA accreditation evaluates how well a health plan manages all parts of its delivery system—physicians, hospitals, other providers, and administrative services—to continuously improve health care for its members. For health care providers to compete on value, they have to provide information on performance and outcomes.

NCQA reviews are rigorous on-site and off-site evaluations conducted by a team of physicians and managed care experts. A national oversight committee of physicians analyzes the team's findings and assigns an accreditation level based on the plan's performance compared with NCQA standards.

These standards—developed by employers, unions, and health plans—are demanding. NCQA has purposely set the standards high to encourage health plans to continuously enhance the quality of health care they deliver. No comparable evaluation exists as yet for fee-for-service health care (that is, the traditional health care structure we were all familiar with).

One level of accountability is provided by the Health Plan Employer Data and Information Set (HEDIS). HEDIS attempts to define and standardize the measurement process for NCQA. HEDIS allows purchasers to follow a yearly trend to compare health plans. The five areas include quality of care, member access, membership and utilization, finance, and descriptive information. As HEDIS has become the benchmark in performance, it has also become helpful for accountability purposes.

HEDIS 2.0, released in 1993, is a set of 60 performance measures for managed care plans and has undergone one technical update (HEDIS 2.5). HEDIS has become the industry standard—it contains the underlying data used to create most health plan "report cards"— and is currently used by more than 330 health plans nationwide, either for their own quality improvement efforts or because purchasers with whom they do business require the reporting of HEDIS data.

One of the primary goals of HEDIS 3.0, currently being developed, is to create a measurement set that is more responsive to the needs of the people covered by Medicare and Medicaid. HEDIS 3.0 is being designed to respond to consumer (patient) and purchaser (insurer or employer) interest in health plan quality. These measures of outcomes are intended to further NCQA ability to provide consumers with the information they need to make meaningful decisions about which health care plan to choose.

Which HMO Has the Patient's Best Interests at Heart?

The patient does not traditionally come first in the HMO industry, because the employer often pays the bill. The company wants the best care for the price. The patient wants the best care. By the end of 1996 approximately 56 million people will have signed up with almost 600 HMOs.

There is no shortage of opinions as to how to pick the best HMO, but the truth is that nobody knows yet. No rating system exists. The report cards that do exist have proved so unhelpful that a group of large employers teamed up with the Health Care Financing Administration (HCFA) to form the Foundation for Accountability.

Since the issue of health care is so complex, the Foundation started with a simple definition: Good health care is the way you would like members of your family to be treated in sickness and in health. Cost was not particularly relevant to their quest. Therefore, looking at basic measures to answer the quality patient care question, they established the following benchmarks:

- Full NCQA accreditation. The sooner it is received, the higher the score.
- Not-for-profit status. Decisions based on patient welfare come first.
- Medical loss ratio. What portion of each dollar received is spent on patient care?
- Compensation. The most points went to HMOs with physicians on salary.
- Turnover. A stream of arriving and departing doctors is disruptive to the patient.
- Certification. A higher percentage of board-certified physicians ranks higher.
- Disenrollment rate. Voluntary and involuntary disenrollment is measured.

Accreditation status is not a guarantee of the quality of care that any individual patient will receive or that any individual physician or other provider will deliver. However, not-for-profit plans that are accredited early with salaried, board-certified physicians, a high medical loss ratio, low turnover rate, and low disenrollment rate demonstrate superior patient-focused standards. And those that closely monitor their performance and strive for continuous improvement rank highest for the quality of care they deliver.

Lessons Learned From Other Projects

It is imperative that the patient remain alert to each of the many steps in the diagnostic, treatment, and healing process and discuss the effect of actions taken today on events tomorrow. Treating a life-threatening disease can be grueling and requires sustained effort. Not only does it change the patient's view of life, it sets forth new ground rules for living.

In project management one seeks to plan, organize, coordinate, execute, and control a series of interlocking events with the goal of reaching a desired result. If you have ever held a job or run part or all of a business, you will quickly recognize the fundamentals.

"The devil is in the details," goes the old saying. The key to running a successful enterprise is in staying on top of the details. Farming counts on time, weather, and constant attention. Home improvement relies on materials, tools, and skills. Health care takes skills, experience, time, and healing.

Managing your health care project means overseeing each of the many steps in the treatment and healing process. At some point it may take personal relaxation exercises; at another stage it may call for *positive visualization,* the method used by many champion athletes.

Congratulations! Project managing your own prostate cancer case is your new full-time job. However, keep in mind that few if any undertakings call for the manager to perform all of the respective activities. Building a house, sending a rocket into space, and treating prostate cancer require team effort. The surgeon relies on a skilled team to support the intricate tasks for which he or she has been trained. When your life is on the line you need to learn quickly how to gather and use information to further your project objectives and to make more effective decisions.

Managing Professionals

My career had given me experience in managing professionals and teams of experts. Among these were economists, engineers, planners, lawyers, ecologists, biologists, architects, anthropologists, researchers, and the like. Each professional person functions from a specific frame of reference, which influences the perception of a problem, and, just as an optical lens can clarify or distort information received through the eyes, affects decision making by acting as a filter that sways our expectations and our reading of events. A variety of decision contexts exist, but one particularly important factor is the decision maker's area of professional specialization.

"Dogs come when they are called; cats take a message and get back to you," wrote Mary Bly. Likewise, members of each professional field represent a distinct species and behave in different ways.

These experts provide their services on the premise that professional integrity and training are paramount in the decision process. Unfortunately, a layperson often is at a marked disadvantage when coping with specialized jargon and may become overwhelmed in such a situation. (For this reason, an extensive Glossary has been included.) It is not unknown for health care professionals to rain complicated terms on the patient's head to demonstrate their superior mastery of the subject, thus inadvertently quelling the many questions that may be forming in the patient's mind.

At one point in my career it was necessary for me to manage different teams of attorneys who worked on interrelated cases for my employer. It was vital that arguments in one case not conflict with aspects of another case or the overall effort. Although I am not a lawyer, my job was to keep the teams on track, help them to define the issues, and jointly find the best course of action under uncertain circumstances. The lawyers' job was to understand the legal, business, and social aspects of the case, to recommend a preferred course of action, and, with the client's approval, to pursue it.

Another situation comes to mind. An engineering-scientific team argued strenuously from their distinct points of view about alternate courses of action. A hydrologist (water supply expert) wanted to drill more wells to *supply* more drinking water. A hydrogeologist (underground water expert) argued for fewer wells, strategically spaced to *capture* more groundwater recharged from rainfall. The marine biologist argued for saving natural vegetation to enhance nature's ability to *retain* larger amounts of ground water. Supplying, capturing, and retaining water are all necessary to maintain a natural cycle.

Reflecting on your own background, you can probably recall one or more complex problem in which you took charge to manage the situation until it was resolved. Have you ever had to talk to different mechanics about which course of action would correct a problem in your car? Or coordinated the efforts of the Little League parents to upgrade the team's diamond?

A man cornered me following an American Cancer Society Man to Man meeting. It was shortly after he learned that he now had a dangerously elevated PSA level. His quandary was what to do next. He had already delayed going to a urologist for several weeks. He did not understand what options were available to him. I asked whether he had prior business experience, whether he had worked with accountants or lawyers, who have their own language. He stopped me, realization dawning in his expression, and said, "I guess it is time for me to take charge of my case." Once you resolve to take charge, it seems to be the obvious and familiar course.

You may have other prior experiences at work, at home, on the playing field, or in community activities. The specific events are less important than the seasoning you have already gained. The exercise can now help serve as a model as you start to take charge of your health situation. Taking charge of my prostate cancer case was far and away the most important assignment of my life. And it was too important to be delegated solely to health care professionals, despite their competence. There was a need for my active participation in all treatment decisions. After all, I was the one who had to live with the results. It soon gave me a wider and deeper appreciation of the potential benefits stemming from forging a strong patient-physician bond.

The Big Assignment

As I have mentioned, with my family background it was certainly not a total shock when I received word that all indicators pointed to prostate cancer; to me it had always seemed more a question of when. Yet in the absence of any real physical symptoms (I thought), and following on the heels of the family doctor's DRE and his reassuring statements, it struck me that just possibly the initial finding might be in error.

I did not know much about the prostate gland, but I was soon to learn more than I ever imagined about the subject. First, I read that the normal prostate is about the size and shape of a walnut. (In a small boy, the prostate is about the size of an almond.) Through the center runs the urethra, the tube that carries urine from the bladder out through the penis. When the prostate becomes enlarged, as it does naturally as part of the male aging process, the urethra may become squeezed, causing a slowing down of urine flow.

I was at the point of choice—to quarterback my own case or let the physician run with management of my treatment plan. How was this dilemma to be reconciled?

Conservative Medicine

Any individual can develop overconfidence that may lead to precipitous action, regardless of his or her occupation, intelligence, or experience. The one factor that has been shown to reduce such overconfidence is feedback. People whose job involves frequent feedback on the accuracy of their decisions, such as weather forecasters, airline pilots, and urologic surgeons, become more realistic in calibrating their own performance. Their self-confidence has a basis in fact.

Over the years it had been my sense that conservative medicine is the best medicine. When Suzi was expecting our children, her pregnancies were somewhat difficult. Her obstetrician was careful to avoid prescribing medications unnecessarily and advised her to limit travel. The pediatrician routinely delayed prescribing antibiotic medications unless the illness absolutely demanded it. My own previous illnesses had been treated step by step.

Surgery has been singled out for special concern. In recent years it has come to light that as many as 25% of all bypass operations were unjustified. Radical mastectomies are less frequently performed today than previously, and lumpectomies and radiation therapy are utilized more often. And stereotactic breast examinations, a technologic advance drawn from the NASA space program, is gradually replacing the more invasive breast biopsy. Hysterectomy has been high on the list of surgical excesses. The National Institutes of Health determined that more than 20% of the hysterectomies performed were unnecessary. In the 1980s a U.S. Senate subcommittee found that half of Medicare-covered costs for pacemaker implants were unwarranted. Studies of upper gastrointestinal tract endoscopies have had similar findings.

Problems have also arisen when medications are overprescribed or when they are not properly monitored by a physician. Unnecessary or prolonged use, disregard for their effect in combination with other medications, or failure to test individual patients for an inability to tolerate a drug can occur. The wise physician is always aware of the contraindications to medications, as reported in the *Physician's Desk Reference* or similar source materials. The wise physician also checks with patients frequently for evidence of side effects. Problems of potential addiction with certain tranquilizers, and painkillers especially, are singled out for special surveillance.

Over time, physicians and surgeons have learned that the basic design of the human body is not faulty or capricious, that not everything for which a specific purpose cannot be found has to come out or be irradiated, and that most people can coexist quite satisfactorily with their own organs, including in most cases the appendix and tonsils. People have gained a new respect for the wisdom of the body.

During an annual company physical examination some 10 years earlier, I had performed marginally on a series of treadmill stress tests. I didn't pass; I didn't fail. Before I knew it, I found myself headed toward a series of advanced stress tests and further heart tests, culminating in a risky heart catherization diagnostic procedure that proved negative. Later, my family doctor shared extensive literature with me pointing up the high incidence of false positive readings in men taking treadmill exercise stress tests. As was eventually proved in my case, this too was a case of the wrong conclusion from the evidence at hand.

Unfortunately, I did not talk with my family doctor first, nor was I aware of advice counseling the patient to take charge of his or her own health care as if it were an assignment. Certainly there was no shortage of "how to" books, but none seemed to stress the need for the patient to *take charge* and actively *participate* in the entire process.

Consequently, I did not pursue the matter early enough, nor did I seek a second opinion from my own family doctor. After all, he knew my physical condition and case better than the internist who was administering the company examination. Motionless, I allowed the physician members of the annual physical examination team to take over all of the important decisions without my first becoming an informed patient, including allowing the examining doctor to call all of the shots. Out of fear, or ignorance, or both, I assumed a passive involvement in the review and decision process. With the opposite approach I might have concluded, before the event, that this dangerous procedure was wholly unnecessary. Time was to bear this out.

When I was younger, I was not as assertive as I am today, lacking the requisite chutzpah. If I had followed the project management approach to health care from the outset, I would have taken three key actions before I agreed to a battery of tests. I would have vigorously reviewed the literature, I would have sought further consultation from our family physician, and I would have had a face-to-face talk with the referring internist and the cardiologist.

During the diagnostic and early treatment phases of my prostate cancer case, under the pressure of time and the fear of a fatal disease, I again came close to forgetting these hard-earned lessons. I also did not keep in mind the merits of a conservative approach to medical treatment. Good health is serious business. Like life itself, it has to be worked at, and with such efforts it takes on added meaning.

At another Man to Man meeting I overheard a discouraged prostate cancer survivor bitterly complain, "my doctor decided that I should do this." Two things struck me. First, an informed patient and active participant in the decision-making process can avoid reaching the point of disillusionment where it is necessary to look back and blame the physician for the critical decisions. Second, it is preferable that all important decisions and actions be taken by an informed patient-physician team.

Chapter 3

From Routine Day to Survival

An Ordinary Day

Until now my annual physical examinations had been uneventful, notwithstanding the heart catheterization scare. Having recently moved to Jacksonville, Florida, we needed to find a new family doctor. After checking with friends and business acquaintances, a young family practice physician was selected. He seemed to have his medical head on straight, at least at first.

As we settled down to business, we exchanged some routine doctor-patient small talk, followed by a brief review of my medical and family history. I was 6 months overdue for this annual ritual, and I wryly remarked, "Most men take better routine care of their cars than they do their personal health."

It is both unwise and regrettable that preventive health care ranks so low on many men's priority lists. Men think they are bulletproof. In addition, they tend to have an adversarial relationship with their doctor. The big three issues in men's health care are cardiovascular (type A personality, hearty eater), lung cancer (type A, first- and second-hand smoking history), and prostate cancer, a disease that respects neither talent nor intellect, nor power or wealth or athletic prowess. Telly Savalas, age 70, who played Kojak, the tough-guy cop on television with the endearing "Who loves ya, baby?" trademark, was silenced by prostate cancer. Actor Bill Bixby, 59, and rock musician Frank Zappa, 52, complained bitterly just before their deaths that their untreatable advanced prostate cancer might have been found earlier and their lives spared by the simple use of a blood test, an inexpensive and noninvasive PSA blood screening. James Herriott, 78, author of the endearing "All Things Great and Small" books and television series, succumbed to prostate cancer. In early 1996, former French president François Mitterand, 79, lost his long fight with prostate cancer. Former Senator Bob Dole, actor-singer Robert Goulet, comedian Jerry Lewis, and former heavyweight boxing champion George Foreman were each lucky that their disease was detected and treated in time. Retired Army general Norman Schwarzkopf's cancer was found through skilled combination screening. Wall Street financier Michael Milken put up his own $25 million in hopes of accelerating research to cure his late-stage prostate cancer.

African-American men have been found to be especially susceptible to prostate cancer for reasons that are not all together clear. Among the members of this celebrated, nonexclusive club are the Reverend Louis Farrakahn, actor Sidney Poitier, Washington, D.C. Mayor Marion Barry, and SNCC activist Kwame Ture (Stokely Carmichael).

As for sports fans, we are in a league with some big-name stars, including baseball's Stan "the Man" Musial, golfing legend Arnold Palmer, race car champion Richard Petty, the late tennis great Bobby Riggs, and famous jockey Eddie Arcaro.

One of my boyhood heroes was my cousin Jack. He often boasted that he had never been sick a day or gone to a doctor in his life. Jack finished tops in his class, both in high school and college, served as a U.S. Coast Guard officer in World War II, and later became a successful tax attorney and CPA. One day he found himself with the unbearable pain of what he soon learned to be late-stage untreatable prostate cancer. Jack died a painful death in just 6 months.

Prostate cancer is a greatly underrated disease. One man recently described his own uncertain condition in this way: "I could think of a lot worse cancers to have." That may be true from a potential healing standpoint, but neglecting those subtle and early signs of changes in voiding patterns and dodging the annual DRE and PSA test after age 50 (or age 40 if there is a family history of prostate cancer) may invite the unnecessary risk of an untimely death. Norman Schwarzkopf asserts, in his brusque military style, "It is stupid for any man to have to die of this disease!" Prostate cancer is called the silent killer for a good reason.

Carefully Listen for Your Doctor's Interests and Biases

At the time of my annual physical examination, Americans were immersed in a fierce and emotional debate about national health care. Our new family physician spent most of my examination denouncing the Clinton administration's attempts to find methods for providing universal health care for all Americans. He also voiced strong concern about the rising number of malpractice suits. The doctor seemed well armed with all of the arguments.

In between, he checked me over in routine fashion, including administering the DRE, after which he declared, "Everything feels fine, and you seem to be in great shape." I asked him to specifically describe how the prostate felt. He said, "soft and pliable."

Complete blood tests were ordered. I requested that the series include the PSA test. I had first learned of the PSA screening test 18 months earlier from Cynthia, who had heard of it on a television news report. After my annual physical examination that year, we mulled over my going back to ask the doctor to confirm that the PSA had been performed. Mistakenly, after scanning a two-page printout of $500 worth of laboratory test results, we concluded that the test must have been performed. Wrong! I was shocked to learn later that none of my prior annual physical examinations had included this inexpensive test, even though each doctor had taken a medical history, performed the DRE, and supposedly ordered a complete set of blood tests. If I had been more persistent at the time, perhaps my prostate cancer would have been detected before it had progressed to the locally advanced stage.

Ironically, more than 10 years earlier my older brother had had an enlarged prostate that impeded smooth urine flow. He underwent a transurethral resection of the prostate (TURP) procedure, which can be envisioned as something like coring an apple. It removes excess tissue and relieves pressure on the urethra. His results came back from the pathology laboratory as positive, and for 6 weeks he was treated for prostate cancer with a once-a-day bombardment of external beam radiation. Since that time he had been given an annual PSA test to monitor his postoperative situation. For some reason, he had never thought to alert me to the potential importance of PSA screening. His doctor had not made him aware of the genetic link with the disease, and I did not know enough or think enough about it to ask.

Today, when any of my friends or business acquaintances stand still for 2 minutes, they receive my unsolicited pitch on the importance of an annual DRE and PSA blood test. My chiropractor has teasingly dubbed me "the PSA poster boy."

♦ **Taking Charge Advisory 1:** Ask for a *urologist-administered* digital rectal examination (DRE) and prostate-specific antigen (PSA) blood test.

First News—First Decisions

Two days after my physical examination, a nurse called to break the news that my PSA level was 41.8. I was to be referred to a urologist. "What's normal?" I asked the nurse. For my age group, I learned, anything between 0 and 4 is considered acceptable. I should have known that myself! Every man in this age group needs to know these facts.

"You mean I am 37.8 points higher than the highest acceptable number?" I screeched over the phone. (That is more than 10 times the acceptable limit, I thought to myself.) My simple math calculation was quickly scored correct. Nonetheless, the nurse could not, or would not, provide any further information.

Why hadn't the doctor called to "break the news" and to brief me on what comes next? With no word from him and little to go on, I felt as though I were teetering at the edge of the abyss, and I expected the worst.

What Does This Mean? What Happens Next?

Shortly thereafter, the doctor called and apologized for not having taken the time to reach me himself. I asked, "What does this mean? What happens next?" He only repeated what the nurse had relayed to me. I was being referred to a urologist. He did not and would not discuss it further.

In retrospect, perhaps he did not want to alarm
more to this? Could he possibly scare me more tha
few days later Cynthia and I ran into the doctor
Normally an outgoing, talkative kind of guy, suddenly stan....
to face with me, he looked almost stunned and definitely uncomfortable, and too unnerved to talk to us. From a perspective of more than
2 years, I can see events more clearly and imagine his thought
processes. Here was a patient on whom he had performed a DRE and
given the prostate a clean bill of health, clearly missing the essential
characteristics that would soon be confirmed by a urologist: a twice-
normal-size prostate with the hardening and lumpy nodular growth
that signaled trouble, as confirmed by my significantly elevated PSA
level.

He assured me that he had never had a PSA result that was a "bad
actor." (What did that mean?) It seemed to me that he was offering an
unrealistic expectation, a false reassurance to assuage his discomfort.
I no longer was left teetering—I now felt as though a large trap door
had been opened and I was being asked to step through and take my
chances in free fall.

Initial Information

With a rapidly beating heart, I called a personal friend and our
former family physician, Dr. Barry Poliner, who practices in another
city. He took the call immediately, recognized what the indicators in
my case probably meant, and clearly laid out what the next diagnostic steps would most likely involve. The call to Dr. Poliner once again
reminded me that there are physicians who care for their patients and
welcome them as team members. For the moment, simply knowing
what was to come next helped set my mind at ease. Not that the news
was likely to be good, but rather, I could better understand and monitor the actions the specialist would probably be taking. It looked as
though I had better get educated fast.

One of the most bewildering and frightening experiences a patient can have is the helplessness that is felt as he or she is passed
along in the health care process, not knowing or understanding what
is about to happen. Few things are more delicate or important in dealing with serious illness than the psychological environment in which

patient is treated. If the physician communicates a serious diagnosis in a way that produces feelings of despair in the patient, the result can sometimes have a negative effect on the course of the disease.

Scientific evidence now exists proving that depression, a common response to a diagnosis of a serious disease, can actually compromise the effectiveness of the disease-fighting capacity of the individual's immune system. Therefore the artistry of the physician in communicating a diagnosis can help get the most out of medical treatment.

Most physicians are probably not insensitive to the emotional needs and responses of patients in the way they communicate their findings, but the economic incentives run in the wrong direction. Medical plans do not compensate physicians for taking the time to talk to their patients. An even more basic factor in "cold turkey communication" of bad news is perhaps that the physician is worried about malpractice suits. Doctors have been conditioned by lawyers and malpractice insurance carriers. Lawyers want certainty, patients want change and improvement in their condition, and physicians are caught in the middle.

Unfortunately, lawyers have also indoctrinated physicians to believe that it is wrong to leave any doubts in the patient's mind about negative possibilities. If anything can go wrong, the lawyers generally recommend that the patient not be surprised. This has led some physicians to tell the patient the worst (or paradoxically in other cases, to say nothing at all) to protect themselves.

Compassion, personal interest, and artistry in communication are more than just essential skills. They are probably the best insurance policy against lawsuits that a physician can acquire. They also help create an environment in which the special abilities of the physician can be shown to greatest advantage.

It seemed a good time to verify my PSA results as I slid along the slippery slope toward a definitive diagnosis. What facts did I have? First, I was asymptomatic (or so I thought) and felt pretty good, although a little more tired. Second, my doctor had assured me that by DRE my prostate felt fine (that is, negative).

I went back to the family doctor's office and asked that my blood be drawn again and this time be sent to two different laboratories for PSA evaluation. I wanted to confirm the initial test findings. The PSA test results would now serve as the foundation on which all bricks would be stacked.

Not surprisingly, there was a terrible gnashing of teeth in the doctor's office over such an unorthodox request from a patient. Recently I learned from news reports that a laboratory had misread two Pap smear tests and that both young women prematurely succumbed to cervical cancer. Testing for cancer is not like checking for a malfunctioning computer chip, yet some health care professionals look on tests as simple or routine, when in fact cancer screening is anything but foolproof. Since it was my life on the line and my dollars being spent to repeat the tests, I wondered why all the fuss?

Finally, after getting my way, I innocently asked the receptionist how they selected the laboratory that performed the initial PSA test. Her response stunned me. "It's the cheapest," she cheerfully chirped back. The office manager overheard this and jumped in with alarm, reassuring me that quality, not cost, was the determining factor in their selection of the laboratory. As I left the office with an amused but disquieted feeling, I thought to myself, "This doctor has good reason to worry about malpractice."

♦ **Taking Charge Advisory 2:** If in doubt, verify the results.

The Referral

With only the name and number of a complete stranger, I phoned the urologist for an appointment and was promptly told that I needed to wait 2 weeks since the doctor was leaving shortly for vacation. Everyone is entitled to rest and rehabilitation but, because I am a mostly type A personality, I slowly and pointedly spelled out the fact that my PSA count was 41.8 and, given the fact that the initial PSA test was so far outside the acceptable range, I wanted to see the urologist that week or be referred to another urologist. Suddenly, miraculously, an appointment was set—I was to be there in 2 hours. Whatever else one believes, the practice of medicine is still a business.

The Booklets

After a brief DRE, the urologist delivered his noticeably canned explanation of what he felt, a hardness on one side, and what this might mean—the likelihood that it was prostate cancer. He was uncertain whether the cancer might have already spread outside of the gland. Only 3 days earlier the family doctor had declared that the prostate he felt was soft and normal. Now seemed like a good time to start feeling alarmed and confused. What other news lay in store?

Some prostate cancer booklets, furnished by one of the pharmaceutical companies, were handed to me. One was dog-eared and most of the information seemed standardized, jargon-heavy, and terribly out of date. Arrangements were made for me to have an outpatient ultrasound examination and biopsy when the doctor returned from vacation.

On the next stop in this new odyssey, I walked over to the hospital scheduling department. I headed straight for the information desk in the main lobby, which was packed with people. I was shunted over to preregister for outpatient services. Name, social security number, and body part were logged into the computer. Appointment time and place to be were designated. I was handed two bottles of some awful-looking stuff, dutifully given instructions for drinking it, wished well in a rather programmed manner, and then aimed toward the exit.

Evaluating a hospital starts by assessing its people and how they deal with patients. There was little doubt that this hospital, one of the largest in the city, had all of the requisite high-tech equipment, physicians, and staff. But a hospital is only a building. The episodes with hospital administrative and support personnel were a foreshadowing of my soon-to-come diagnostic ordeal.

Hospital or health care administration is a demanding field calling for a variety of intensively trained individuals. Managers oversee a variety of people who are expected to be highly skilled. This is the professional side of the equation.

A more subjective way of assessing hospital facilities is to tour them. This can be arranged through the hospital public information office. In my early experience as an ethical drug representative, I had many times walked the corridors of a hospital. I have always assessed the following:

- Is the building clean and in good repair?
- Is equipment stored properly and not left unprotected in public areas such as corridors?
- Does security control traffic and access so unauthorized people are not wandering around?
- Are the staff members busy, and do they appear to be working with intent and organization?
- Is the staff knowledgeable, courteous, and helpful?

Ask for a tour of your hospital. While an on-site visit may not yield a great deal of objective data, you will undoubtedly come away with an overall impression of the hospital, which can be translated into comfort or discomfort as a patient.

Surviving Hospital Tests

A few days later the second and third PSA test results came back and confirmed the initial finding. That meant the urologist's return-from-vacation bonus was to find me waiting on a hospital outpatient table at the appointed time.

A technician performed the ultrasound examination and told me that I could leave immediately after my "pictures" were taken. I hastily pointed out that a biopsy was also scheduled, which I had now come to learn is the essential first-level test for determining whether there is cancer in the prostate gland. As though a badminton birdie were softly floating across a net, we delicately argued the difference between what the scheduling computer showed and my understanding of what was scheduled. Finally, while still lying on my back, I asked that she call my urologist and clear up this mess. Within 15 minutes the doctor arrived to get the rest of the show on the road.

Although hospital administrative staff had processed me promptly, politely, and routinely, they had neglected to schedule the key test—the biopsy. Circumstances such as this reinforced my determination to keep closer tabs on my own case.

This experience alone should help drive home the point. *You need to learn all you can as early as you can about your condition and its treatment.* What tests, drugs, and procedures will be used? What does the doctor want to learn from them? How will this information influence your health care? The answers to these questions will be of vital importance to you.

Table Talk—The Patient Is Listening

The urologist-radiologist team proceeded with the biopsy while I remained awake but with no anesthetic, either local or general. This procedure was in fact fairly uncomfortable. Nonetheless, the doctors jauntily chatted about their respective vacations, seemingly oblivious to the fact that it was a person they were working on. It seemed as though this procedure was interrupting their morning coffee break. Wide awake, I anxiously listened for every nuance and remark that might relate to this very delicate and personal procedure they were performing.

A doctor's off-hand attitude sends signals of disinterest to the patient. The result is neither comforting nor reassuring. The biopsy was physically painful. Although the procedure was clearly a routine matter to the team, its results were to determine a potentially life-threatening diagnosis for me.

At one time doctors assumed that because patients undergoing surgery were usually sedated or anesthetized, it really didn't matter what they talked about, but today there is ample evidence that this is not so. Studies document that under hypnosis patients can recall statements made during surgery by the operating team. Hypnosis and ventilation therapy have been used successfully to treat unexplained postoperative anxiety and depression attributable to remarks made during surgery. At the Second National Conference on the Psychology of Health, Immunity and Disease in 1990, participants were reminded that patients under anesthesia are not asleep—they are unconscious. When they are unconscious, their auditory system is still active, and even though they do not consciously remember what is heard, they can still learn. (This phenomenon is confirmed by the long success with sleep tapes by some people.) A commentator at the conference warned, "The real issue is, what is learned during surgery persists later but is not identified by the patient as resulting from the operative period." Therefore health care providers bear responsibility for using this time as an opportunity to provide therapeutic messages and healing comments for patient recovery.

After collecting only three of the requisite six tissue snips from my prostate, the urologist looked at the monitor screen with me and explained the location of the prostate and the areas of probable trouble. The next diagnostic steps were laid out for me in the most likely event that the pathology laboratory report proved positive, thus confirming the worst—cancer. I was slated to have both a CT scan and a bone scan to detect any spread of the disease. I came to learn much later that these diagnostic steps are not always needed.

Three days later the urologist personally phoned to go over the pathology findings, which were positive, meaning cancer was found. Further, the pathology laboratory had determined that my cell growth was poorly differentiated—which meant a nonuniform cell pattern with rapid growth. A well-differentiated cell structure follows a pattern of replacing good or healthy cells with the same configuration of cancerous cells. In prostate cancer, 85% of the time well-differentiated cell growth is the more common finding and generally signals a slow growth phenomenon. On the other hand, poorly differentiated cells mean the cancer cells are growing in a bizarre arrangement with continuous branching—the most rapidly growing and virulent form of the disease. The bone and CT scans were scheduled to determine whether there were any signs of spreading to other sites in my body. Sweat beads now formed all over my brow.

I traveled back to the hospital outpatient department to preregister for the new series of radiology scan tests. This brought me face to face with the same schedulers. Vital statistics and tests were logged in and two bottles of ominous-looking liquid were dispensed, accompanied by cryptic instructions as to when and how much of this stuff to drink and some maladroit best wishes.

Several days later, at the appointed time and place, the radiology desk nurse asked me to drink one of the two bottles of liquid given to me by scheduling. As I removed the bottle from the paper bag, the nurse glanced at it and shouted with alarm, "Don't drink that!" This time, I had been given the wrong liquid!

Vigilance takes energy. Remember, you are the paying client, and health care is a purchased service. The patient needs to be encouraged to be knowledgeable and to speak up.

Having narrowly escaped another close call with hospital bureaucracy and the support staff's performance, I went home to await another call from my urologist. Both the CT scan and bone scans were clear! For the moment my sweat dried.

This was our first celebrative experience. Cynthia and I had been understandably scared and worried. We were now greatly relieved that the cancer had not already traveled beyond the prostate capsule to metastasize elsewhere in my body. More than a few tears of joy flowed freely that evening. I was soon to learn, however, that we were still far from the finish line.

Dire Consequences Conference

It was time to meet with the urologist to learn by way of charts and explanations the alternative courses of action in my case. Being a surgeon, he strongly recommended surgical removal of the prostate, a radical prostatectomy, and the sooner the better. He also said that it was possible that radiation therapy might be necessary postoperatively in a case such as mine.

The doctor was critical of using any form of radiation treatment alone and thought that in this situation, there was no other course of action than a radical prostatectomy. He stressed that the disease was too serious and, at my age (61), it was also growing too fast for watchful waiting (in which the care provider performs no aggressive treatment and waits to see whether the condition progresses) or, especially, to be neglected. He spoke frankly about the amount of discomfort to be expected with a radical prostatectomy, describing it as a deep punch in the gut, and the postoperative side effects that I might expect. He outlined an 8-day hospital stay, to be followed by 6 to 8 weeks of at-home recuperation. I was encouraged to solicit matching blood donors and, together with autologous donation (blood given by the donor for his own eventual use), to stockpile 4 to 6 pints of blood.

Down at the blood bank an entire fraternity (and sorority) of donors met regularly, and I found a new group of folks with whom to exchange war stories. The radical prostatectomy procedure is very invasive. In the hands of surgeons of differing skills, the results may differ. I was later to learn that a usage of 2 pints was more typical.

Several times during our talk, the subject of merits of obtaining a second opinion came up. The doctor insisted that he had no objection and strongly encouraged patients to seek another opinion. However, in my case, he emphasized, the cancer was of a very aggressive type and under no circumstances should I delay obtaining aggressive treatment. He gave no indication that the cancer might have already spread outside of the prostate capsule. He hastened to point out that in circumstances such as mine, at the Mayo Clinic, also located in Jacksonville, they routinely performed a bilateral orchiectomy—the surgical removal of the testes. That certainly caused me to sit up straight and pay closer attention! Only later would I come to see the gross inconsistencies in what this urologist was telling me.

It was increasingly clear that the point of no return was rapidly approaching and it was ever more urgent that I learn everything possible about the diagnosis and treatment of prostate cancer. Certainly, I needed to know much more than I knew at that moment.

Prostate cancer had become a very involved subject indeed. I was heading for an admittedly very invasive procedure, a promised long hospital stay, probably multiple blood transfusions, a long and uncomfortable recovery period, an almost certain need for postoperative radiation therapy, uncertainty about whether the interventions would be a total success, and the potential for the permanent side effects of incontinence, impotence, or both. At this point, all I had to go on was the advice of a urologist in a one-physician office. I had met him only twice. I had been referred by a family physician who I hardly knew and who had already chalked up one major blunder.

Notwithstanding the continued uncertainty, one thing now seemed clear enough. I had little choice but to move forward quickly with some decision while I increased my knowledge. Surgery was scheduled for 1 month from that day.

♦ **Taking Charge Advisory 3:** Don't delay treatment decisions.

Leaving the urologist's office, it was altogether clear that what was needed was more than a second opinion. The issues were more complex, grave, and far reaching than I had earlier expected, and more was at stake than just following this doctor's advice.

I was now fully aware that I had a very serious case of prostate cancer—that a time bomb was ticking away inside my body. The countdown toward surgery had started, and with it my intensive search for new information.

Over the next 3 weeks my blood bank account was built, and I systematically revisited and questioned each step taken or considered thus far:

- What do I know about this urologist?
- How can I learn about treatment options in my case?
- Would a second opinion be of any value at this late stage? If so, how?
- Are the multiple mistakes made at the hospital a red flag?
- Where do I turn for sufficient information on which to base a decision this late in the game?
- Are the warnings about the Mayo Clinic of genuine concern, or was the urologist an alarmist?

I had to conclude that a health care system that functions primarily with its own purposes and goals in mind can never be expected to deliver a superior level of patient care. There was little doubt that my confidence index with this hospital and its administrative staff had steadily fallen, even though it was one of the most prominent health centers in this city. As for the urologist, my mind remained open while my gut signaled otherwise. I further concluded the following:

- The family doctor, at best, cared about me as a customer.
- Some hospital staff members had repeatedly shown that they lacked proper diligence.
- The diagnosing urologist showed only routine regard toward my case.
- To date, all players practiced "body part" medicine.

At this point I summed it up this way: Neither the doctors and their staff nor the hospital staff really cared for me as a person. They had made no effort to know the person who was about to undergo life-threatening, invasive surgery and eventual protracted recovery. They had not asked, who is this man? Does he have a family? What could he accomplish with an extended life span? Can I empathize with his fears and concerns?

Sir William Osler, famed medical professor, once noted: "It is more important to know what sort of person this disease has than to know what sort of a disease this person has."

I shared my personal misgivings about the hospital with the diagnosing urologist, specifically, the hospital's repeated simple mistakes and the rather impersonal nature of this particular corner of the health care system. His response was honest, but unsettling. "I can't speak for the health care system," he quipped. Each day the reality came closer that my life would be in his hands and in the arms of this hospital. Finally, I asked myself whether this was the best team to deliver emotional support, that intangible aspect of health care so necessary to hope and healing, to me and my family?

The surroundings of medical testing and care, including the attitudes and manner of the caregivers, carry more weight in the outcome for the patient than is generally recognized by busy and hard-pressed medical staffs. And the value of the patient-physician relationship continues to grow in significance.

The part played by the human mind and spirit in healing has been well documented. In *Love, Medicine & Miracles*, Dr. Bernie Siegel counsels, "Getting well is not the only goal. Even more important is learning to live without fear, to be at peace with life and death." In *Head First*, Norman Cousins wrote about patient attitudes toward cancer: "More than 90% of the physicians said they attach the highest value to attitudes of hope and optimism." Dr. William J. Mayo, cofounder of the Mayo Clinic, summed it up this way: "The best interest of the patient is the only interest to be considered."

Chapter 4

A Statistical Case of One

Men, Screening, and Denial

Only a small number of prostate cancer cases are detected solely by DRE. However, when the DRE is done by a skilled urologist and a PSA blood test is obtained, the detection rate for prostate cancer rises significantly.

The reported infrequency with which the DRE is performed on patients is somewhat startling. In a screening program of 433 men over age 40 conducted at the Cleveland Clinic between 1989 and 1990, the information clearinghouse Patient Advocates for Advanced Cancer Treatments, Inc. (PAACT) reported that two thirds of the men said they had not had a DRE performed during the previous year. Even more unsettling is the fact that of about 150 who reported having a general physical examination in the prior year, a DRE was performed on less than 60% of these patients. The reasons cited for why men fail to get a DRE screening for prostate cancer include the following:

- Since early-stage cancers cannot be felt, there is no need for it.
- The DRE is repulsive—not a macho thing.
- A doctor probing their rectum is distasteful.
- The risks of prostate cancer if not detected early are not known.
- Financial resources or access to screening facilities are limited.
- A diagnosis of cancer of a sexually related gland is frightening.

The prognosis (chance of recovery) and the choice of treatment depend on the stage of the cancer. Once cancer has been diagnosed, more tests are done to determine the extent to which the disease may have spread to other tissues of the body. This is called *staging* the disease.

I continued to review the facts that determine clinical staging to sharpen my appreciation of how different stages of prostate cancer develop and how the diagnosis in my particular case stood in the hierarchy of the disease. Eventually, the ability to appreciate subtle differences in staging and treatment success rates would prove to be the key to fully understanding the potential effectiveness of alternate treatments in my particular case. To further refine my decision process, I matched different prostate cancer stages with the most common treatments for each stage. This mix-and-match exercise forced me to sift through a stack of clinical trial reports and technical findings. Later, it would all come together to help answer the crucial question—Which treatment?

Staging and Gleason Scores

A brief summary of the old and new systems of staging appears below. A more complete definition of each stage is included in Appendix C (also see the Glossary). Most important is that the implications, as related to your particular case, should be *understood* and *thoroughly reviewed* with your physician.

Stages of Prostate Cancer

Old System (Whitmore-Jewett)	New System (TNM)	Characteristics
A	T1	Confined to prostate; detected by DRE unexpectedly
B	T2	Confined to prostate; detected by DRE or ultrasonography
C	T3	Locally advanced beyond prostate
D	N+ or M+	Spread to pelvic lymph nodes (N+) or distant organs (M+)

If the disease is diagnosed when it is confined to the prostate and is treated promptly, a cure generally can be achieved. If the disease has spread to the bones, the average survival is only about 3 years, even with the best available treatments, although there have recently been reports of some longer survival periods. In any event, the difference points up the vital importance of early diagnosis.

At one Man to Man support group meeting, several of us compared our Gleason scores. Shockingly, but perhaps not too surprisingly, one man said he had been fighting prostate cancer for more than 4 years and did not have the foggiest notion what we were all talking about. I don't think you can know too much about a disease that can cost you your life.

♦ **Taking Charge Advisory 4:** Find out what it all means.

Individual Research—Weighing the Options

With less than a month to go before my date with the surgeon's knife, it was vital to fold any new information into my thinking, to integrate the notes and articles already collected. In this way any reasonable alternative that still remained open could be taken into account.

The treatment choices for prostate cancer offer two routes—the traditional pathway and the nontraditional pathway. With the traditional pathway the options come down to the choice between two standard treatments: a radical prostatectomy or external beam radiation. Nonstandard treatments such as cryosurgery, seed implantation, hypothermia, and combination hormonal therapy were largely unfamiliar to me at the time.

There are several advantages to traditional treatments over nonstandard treatments that need to be considered:

1. Ten-year survival statistical studies are available. These can provide some degree of comfort and confidence.
2. Traditional treatments are considered less risky in terms of survival. Simply, more is known about them.
3. More trained physicians practice traditional treatments. In the game of chance, the patient's odds of success are improved.
4. More hospitals provide traditional treatments. There is less likelihood of error resulting from unfamiliar circumstances.
5. Most insurance companies are prepared to reimburse for traditional procedures. The system is set up to handle the routine situations.

With not much time left until surgery day, Cynthia and I went to the bookshop to load me up with reading material for the hospital stay and to also help keep me busy during the expected 6- to 8-week recuperation period. I browsed the magazine rack for mind-numbing stuff—cars, computers, or business. Cynthia, bless her heart, read the prostate cancer books.

We sat together on a bench to peruse what she l
the same old stuff. Suddenly, we came across an
heading, "How to Select a Doctor." Like most patien
that referral to a specialist from a family doctor was
But our new family doctor had already proved to ᴗe a disappoint-
ment. We continued to read.

The first line stopped us in our tracks. Very straightforward and
simple it read, "Determine whether your surgeon is board certified."
Determine whether your surgeon is board certified, I repeated out loud.
DETERMINE WHETHER YOUR SURGEON IS BOARD CERTIFIED!
The words shouted from the page.

Pushing Forward to Get the Facts

I did not have the slightest idea whether my urologist was board
certified or not. "Naw," I thought to myself. "He must be board certified. Otherwise the family doctor would not have made the referral."
I needed to know two things and fast. First, *why* is board certification
considered important? Second, is *my* urologist board certified?

A physician who is board certified, I quickly learned, has at least
the minimum proper training in his or her specialty and has demonstrated proficiency through supervision and testing. While there are
many non-board-certified doctors who are highly competent, it is
more difficult to assess the level of their training. Although board certification alone does not guarantee competence, it is a standard that
reflects successful completion of an appropriate training program. It
also helps ensure a basic level of competence (see Appendix D for a
toll-free number to verify board certification).

A telephone search was started first thing in the morning to find
the answers. First, the consulting nurse with my health insurance carrier honestly expressed her personal preferences but confirmed that
insurance reimbursement would not be affected. Next, a call went out
to the Chief of Urology at the hospital where I was already scheduled
to have surgery. He confirmed that inasmuch as the hospital permit-
ted the doctor an affiliation and extended surgical privileges, it indicated that the hospital's measure of competence had been met. He
further hastened to offer a second opinion, if there was still some concern. Then I confronted the urologist directly. He acknowledged that
he was not board certified. He had sat for his boards, failed them, and
then his practice had gotten too busy for him to retake the examination.

I went back to directly challenge the referring family doctor, who panicked when I confronted him with the question of the urologist's board qualifications. He seemed genuinely surprised and quickly assured me that he had been totally unaware that the doctor to whom I had been referred was not board certified in urology. He offered to make another referral, which at this point seemed about as reliable as my just scanning the yellow pages. Finally, I innocently asked him, "Why did you choose this particular doctor for my referral?" I was floored by his answer. "Because he was conveniently located," he said.

Patients Learn the New Rules

Years ago, patients took the words of the doctor as law or as gospel—not to be questioned, maybe not even discussed. That is not the case today. Consumers are better informed about health issues and need to be actively involved in the decision making that affects their health. Yet some patients do not feel this need and are comfortable accepting a medical diagnosis or course of treatment without question. Some doctors—thankfully, in diminishing numbers—feel uncomfortable with patients who want everything explained to them or want to be involved in the decision making. Consider how you feel about this issue and discuss it openly with your doctor to be certain you are on the same wavelength.

A patient care model based on patient ignorance is unlikely to survive today's information-rich environment. Increasingly, patients will not only read all the literature available in the popular press but will also use the power of on-line computer services and the Internet to tap into patient resources, medical libraries, and databases. They will discuss ailments and experiences with other survivors who are network users and then follow diagnostic decision trees. Consequently, the best patient treatment model for the future is one that assumes that patients will come to know as much as their doctors—not about how to practice medicine, but about what medical practice has to offer.

◆ **Taking Charge Advisory 5:** Broaden your search.

Sharing the News With Others

I started to discuss my personal situation with friends and colleagues. By coincidence, a bit of providence, or both, three important events soon converged to change the course of my activities.

First, it turned out that an old friend, Lou Steflik, had learned 6 months earlier that he too had prostate cancer. Lou is a retired farmer who had for many years raised cabbages and potatoes in a small rural Florida county. Research has shown that farmers exhibit a higher than average incidence of prostate cancer. It is suspected that this may have something to do with the long-term use of agricultural fertilizers and chemicals. Since learning of his disease, Lou had traveled to different hospitals and specialists trying to decide which course of treatment to select, and he also struggled with the decision about which doctor to select.

Lou and I and our wives lunched together. We guys talked prostate cancer; the women talked about what would come next. Lou shared a thick file folder of articles with me that he had accumulated on the subject. He talked about something about which I had not yet heard: a nerve-sparing radical procedure pioneered by Dr. Patrick Walsh at Johns Hopkins, a surgical method with a reportedly high success rate in avoiding postoperative impotence. Lou had already been evaluated at a leading teaching hospital but remained uncertain whether the surgeon who would perform his particular surgery would be instructing or performing the surgery himself. He had gone to a local urologist, a long-time friend, who assured him that he would use the nerve-sparing procedure if at all possible.

Lou's original priorities put retaining postoperative sexual prowess high on his list, right up there with survival. Later, his priorities changed when he learned his case had turned out to be more advanced than at first thought. The clincher was that his urologist friend discouraged him from going to Mayo Clinic Jacksonville and did not seem to have a high opinion of Mayo Clinic's urology department.

A Personal Turning Point

I relate the lunch with Lou because of its importance as a turning point for me. Our conversation opened my eyes to the fact that there was still a good deal about prostate cancer I did not know. And it opened my mind to taking more responsibility—to take charge of more events in hopes of ensuring the best results possible under these uncertain circumstances.

I immediately stepped up my literature search and sought out others to talk to. I finally opened up to my colleague, Dr. Leon Lessinger, Eminent Scholar in Education Policy and Economic Development, who was to become my collaborator on the medical coaching portion of this book. He has had his own experience with benign prostatic hyperplasia. Although at first I was nervous, I shared my current situation with him—the disappointing experiences with the hospital and early doctors, and my search for more information. "Whose life is it anyway?" I asked rhetorically.

Some time ago, Leon had been referred to the Mayo Clinic Jacksonville to correct a long-standing internal bleeding problem resulting from a complication of previous prostate surgery. He spoke positively about his experiences with the Mayo Clinic, his urologist, and his total satisfaction with the staff and the way his particular case was handled. We talked about the wisdom as well as the value of having a second opinion, especially this late in my game. As usual he encapsulated the situation in a few words, "What have you got to lose?"

My conscience had already been nagging me for several weeks. Every day I would drive along the Butler Expressway, less than 2 miles from my house, passing the gleaming white edifice of one of the world's foremost medical institutions—the Mayo Clinic. Why hadn't I gone there already? Was I afraid the Mayo Clinic was only for special situations? If this wasn't a special situation, then what on earth was?

I wanted to know whether the Mayo Clinic, as a model of integrated family and specialty practice, would really *care for me,* or merely treat me as a body part with a patient ID number. Where else did my decision paralysis come from? With only 14 days left before the scheduled surgery, time was running out. Was it too late for a second opinion?

♦ **Taking Charge Advisory 6:** Change your doctor if necessary.

Bringing in the Family

At the same time, I achieved a major milestone by opening up about this situation with my children (all 30-something). I had always been the strong fatherly type, never wanting to burden the kids with my problems. I recall my parents were the same old country stoic type. This time, something told me I should discuss my quandary with my sons.

Their empathy, their sensitivity, and their maturity simply overwhelmed me. My sons bombarded me with questions. They stood by me, providing strong support. Along with Cynthia, who is the real heroine in this story, I was pushed to dig deeper, farther, and faster.

A strange, lingering doubt continued to hang over me. I continued to wonder, "Can I abandon my doctor?" In retrospect, it now seems like an odd, almost preposterous, question, but at the time the issue loomed large. After all, the first urologist had performed the biopsies, diagnosed the case, explained the traditional alternatives, and had already gone ahead to schedule the date of surgery. Yet there remained this disquieting feeling—one that only later I could properly define.

I strongly recommend patients to get a second opinion. The first thing I would do is select a surgeon who is highly recognized in the field. What happens in surgery is not just the result of the surgeon's skills but also of how the patient *thinks* about the surgery and the confidence the patient brings into the operating room. *You have the power to program yourself for a good result.*

There are studies of patients going into surgery and the difference it made when the patient had high expectations—if the patient looked forward to being liberated from illness rather than being governed by foreboding. A positive mind-set seems to translate into a more favorable outcome.

♦ **Taking Charge Advisory 7:** Get a second opinion.

Chapter 5

Teamwork Pays Off

Two Weeks and Counting

In less than 2 weeks I would be on the operating room table. Blood had been stockpiled; one of my former employees and still a dear friend offered to donate a pint to the account. Such moments show us that reciprocal warm feelings exist unsuspected among friends. Reading materials were assembled. New pajamas had been purchased and packed. My shaving kit was rechecked for essential personal items. I was ready.

Then, on impulse, I telephoned the Mayo Clinic Jacksonville. I explained my short timetable and asked for a second opinion appointment with Dr. Michael J. Wehle, who had successfully solved Leon's persistent problem. This doctor came highly recommended from a man whose judgment and intellect I greatly respected.

The Mayo Clinic was founded in Rochester, Minnesota more than 100 years ago. Today it enjoys world-class status as a coordinated and integrated group practice. The Mayo Clinic has cared for more than 4 million individuals and serves over 300,000 persons per year from around the world in three major locations: Rochester; Scottsdale, Arizona; and Jacksonville, Florida. About 10 years ago, the Mayo Clinic opened the Jacksonville facility. Today there are approximately 200 physicians supported by a large staff and research facilities, and more than 15,000 physicians from around the world have been trained in Jacksonville.

In 1996, *U.S. News & World Report* again ranked the Mayo Clinic among the top two urology departments in the United States, along with Johns Hopkins, and as one of the two best hospitals in the United States in all specialties. The *Journal of Urology* was, until recently, edited by Dr. Joseph Oesterling, a Mayo Clinic urologist. The *Wall Street Journal* cited the Mayo Clinic as a model managed care facility that already practices cost-effective medicine.

Mayo Clinic responded graciously and promptly to my request. An appointment was set for 2 days later. This gave me just enough hours to hustle around to collect my patient records from the family physician, the diagnosing urologist, and the hospital where all of the testing had been done.

Medical records can be requested by and turned over to insurance companies, lawyers, employers, and others without your consent, although you can see them to make certain they contain the proper information. However, getting hold of my own patient records seemed like a journey through a virtual reality red tape machine at the hospital and both doctors' offices. No one seemed the least bit willing to accommodate my urgent request. If anything, each staff member I dealt with seemed a bit put out; my request seemed to interrupt their customary activities. They were not geared to provide *my* records to meet *my* needs—on short notice. Regrettably, health care is not yet patient-centered. It is still first and foremost a professionally staffed, cost-centered business.

♦ **Taking Charge Advisory 8:** When time is of the essence, demand a quick turnaround.

The Second Opinion Team

At the Mayo Clinic it felt as though I were entering a medical center of the twenty-first century. The facilities were attractive and immaculate, like coming into the lobby of a Marriott Hotel rather than a spartan health care clinic. The Mayo Clinic check-in personnel were efficient and courteous—and completely ready for my arrival. It was as though I were the only patient they had that day.

The elevator trip to the third floor seemed endless, although it took only a few seconds. There I was swallowed up by a large waiting room full of relaxed patients. In the midst of this vast institution there seemed to be a quiet calm. A sense of *medical confidence and personal care* permeated the atmosphere. It was unlike any health care experience I had previously encountered. But the real question remained to be answered: Was it just another "body part" factory? My records were collected and a personal health history form was completed. I then settled down to read a copy of *USA Today*.

When I was fresh out of college, my first job was as a medical pharmaceutical detailer. Carrying a large black bag filled with presentation charts, clinical reports, and samples for patient use, I visited eight to ten doctors' offices each day to provide them with the latest information on my company's assortment of prescription-only drugs. In those days, it was common to find piles of back-issue magazines (mostly 5 years old or older) lying around the doctor's waiting room. I was often struck by the seeming correlation between the stage of a physician's thinking and how outdated the reading material was.

Here, however, today's national newspaper was lying there on the table. Still, the thought of changing doctors weighed heavily on my mind. The most common failings cited by patients who have chosen not to go to their previous doctors any longer include the following:

- Doctors who dismiss problems or are not interested in having the patient as a partner in health care. The effect of the physician's evasiveness can be patient anger, fear, and confusion, leading to failure to follow directions and thus failure of treatment.
- Doctors who are never on time. Medical emergencies arise frequently, and appointment-making is an inexact science. But chronic snafus may be a sign of trouble in the office scheduling structure.
- Doctors who cannot diagnose the problem. Some conditions cannot be diagnosed on-the-spot, but an incomplete workup or a doctor who considers only a narrow range of treatment alternatives may overlook a condition that could have been treated earlier.
- Doctors who order too many tests. Sophisticated technology is available and doctors tend to use it. A good patient-physician team uses collaboration to help improve mutual understanding about what tests are essential to a definitive diagnosis.
- Doctors who dissuade you from talking to another doctor, because they may perceive it as questioning their professional abilities.

- Unpleasant office staff. Doctors who do not demand the highest level of performance from their staff send a message about their own ability to diagnose and treat.

Examination and Prognosis

My first Mayo Clinic health care provider interview was with Karen Ryan, a physician's assistant (PA) in the urology department. Karen, garbed in freshly starched white coat, was bright, attractive, and with a pleasant smile and perfectly combed hair. She initially took all of the pertinent information remaining in my head and not already logged in my medical records that I had brought with me. Because I am fairly traditional, this was a totally new event, one that I was not yet sure to be of my liking. But I continued to play along. After all, much more serious matters were on the agenda.

The Mayo Clinic, as in more and more managed care facilities, now makes increasing use of PAs. A PA is licensed to provide medical care in many states. Unlike nurses, they may practice only under the direction and supervision of a doctor. According to an article in the professional journal *Family Practice Management*, these "mid-level providers," as they are called, can handle 80% to 90% of the problems that occasion office visits. The PA has become more of a presence in health care in recent years, especially in medical groups and large clinics. Ultimately the Mayo Clinic urology PA would play a pivotal role in my treatment and eventual healing.

Right on time, the doctor made his entrance, also garbed in a starched white coat. Mike Wehle is a slender, 6-foot tall, young-looking professional with a full head of hair, stylishly thin-rimmed eyeglasses, and a pleasing, relaxed way about him. He got right down to business. He looked over my records, which turned out to be incomplete from the hospital (I should have figured on that by now).

He then had me prepare for the requisite DRE. Immediately, it was apparent that his DRE touch was unlike what I had experienced in previous evaluations. From my vantage point, *which isn't saying much*, it was clear that this guy would settle any arguments about what was going on up there.

During the DRE, the doctor inserts a gloved, lubricated index finger into the rectum to feel the prostate for enlargement, stiffness, hardness, and nodules. This method takes about 30 seconds and may cause some discomfort. However, it is not painful. Even though the entire prostate gland cannot be examined by DRE, a skilled physician can detect any unusual growths on the prostate where a tumor is likely to occur.

At the conclusion of his examination, the doctor excused himself from the room for a couple of minutes. Although I was unable to see him, Cynthia described his facial expression as "very concerned." Whatever it was that he felt on my prostate, we would soon enough learn what it meant.

Our investigations and readings to this point had convinced us that the literature on prostate cancer and various doctors' opinions on this disease are very confusing. It was certainly much more than a matter of staging T1 to T4 or determining a total Gleason score. Prostate cancer, we had come to learn, is an insidious disease that presents a weighty treatment dilemma for the patient and the doctor. The guidance of some specialists in the field has added further to patient confusion. For example:

- Since the advent of the nerve-sparing technique, some urologists have heavily emphasized the preservation of potency, leaving the patient with potentially conflicting objectives: life or sex?
- Some radiation oncologists recommend that their patients 70 years old or older just wait and see, without providing any clear guidelines.
- Some doctors continue to rely solely on the DRE to identify prostate cancer. That was my case during my annual physical examination 18 months earlier, when my cancer might have been detected at an earlier stage.
- Many of the patients at the support group meetings insist that even though they had greatly enlarged prostates (also my situation), their doctors failed to put them on combination hormonal therapy to "debulk" their prostates and make them more manageable for treatment.
- The urologists that I heard speak at American Cancer Society meetings or who have spoken with other members of my family have tended to be cautious and reluctant to consider the merits of a nontraditional treatment for prostate cancer because there are no 5- and 10-year survival studies.

- Reportedly, some doctors fail to properly follow up with patients who have an elevated PSA level. When they do, it may be a year between tests. (There may be no greater argument than this for the patient taking charge and project managing his own health care.)
- Research seems to suggest that many prostate cancers are actually "understaged" during diagnosis. It is reportedly not uncommon for stage T1 or T2 cancer to be upgraded during surgery to a stage T3.
- In other cases, what was originally diagnosed as a low-grade tumor is found during surgery to have spread to the adjacent lymph nodes, at which point surgery is discontinued. The surgeon proceeds with removal of the prostate only after the lymph nodes have been examined by a pathologist under a microscope and found to be clear of cancer.
- Some doctors fail to do their homework, to remain up-to-date on current research findings, and as a result, present stale or only general information to patients. This gripe is frequently voiced at support group meetings, where patients have often become quite knowledgeable.
- Some doctors fail to properly communicate to their prostate cancer patients and demonstrate insensitivity toward them.
- Some doctors fail to be creative in recommending various treatments for prostate cancer to their patients.
- The traditional standard (sometimes called the gold standard) for prostate cancer treatment is the radical prostatectomy. The traditional standard for removing testosterone (the fuel for prostate cancer growth) from the body is bilateral orchiectomy, surgical removal of both testes. Both standards are badly outdated, with new treatments available. However, it is the physician who must break with tradition.

Again, I want to stress that I am not a physician. I have written this story as a prostate cancer survivor. This means that I *am healed, not cured.*

My life depended on gathering up-to-date information, assimilating new knowledge, and strengthening my ability to effectively manage the many decisions yet to be confronted, and so may your life, or that of a loved one. No stronger motivator is needed to arm yourself with as much useful data as possible.

As manager of your own prostate cancer case, you will need to turn massive amounts of detailed data into manageable form and then use that new knowledge as an active member of an effective patient-physician team.

Findings, Implications, and Alternatives

The news was neither all good nor all bad. First, Dr. Wehle found my prostate to be greatly enlarged, much more so than had been disclosed in the two prior examinations. Next, he confirmed that he could feel the cancer and that it had *definitely* broken through to the outside casing of the gland, in fact, to a considerable extent. Third, the size of my prostate (55 grams) and the locally advanced stage of growth made it doubtful that he could successfully get all of it with a knife. The treatment of choice—a radical prostatectomy—would not be sufficient by itself.

It was becoming increasingly difficult to remember that just 6 weeks earlier the family doctor had declared that my prostate *felt normal,* or that only 5 weeks ago the first urologist conveyed his findings that cancer *might* be felt on one side of the prostate gland.

A bit of black humor struck me. Had they all examined the same prostate gland? Obviously, but the *extent* to which each doctor had performed a DRE differed *markedly,* as had now been demonstrated in these varied findings, each of which could have a distinct bearing on my treatment decision.

From the examining table, I could recognize the differences in each physician's technique and the implications of the individual findings were equally significant. The skill and competency of the urologist's touch in DRE in large measure determines the *significance and reliability of the diagnosis.*

A distinct benefit to the patient of obtaining a second opinion is not merely to confirm that prostate cancer is there; its value is derived from being able to grasp the doctor's interpretation of what was felt during the DRE and what the collected data mean. Together, these factors may come to weigh heavily on your treatment selection.

Dr. Wehle leveled with us about the various alternatives and what they meant in my case. Because the cancer had broken through to the outside of the capsule, there was a 50-50 chance that cancer had already spread farther to the adjacent lymph nodes. And even if it had not spread that far, the doctor was almost certain that he probably could not remove it all with the scalpel. This confirmed the likelihood that if I underwent a radical prostatectomy, it probably could not be totally successful and radiation therapy would also be needed.

Where did this leave me? For the moment it was T3 disease, and too far locally advanced for a radical procedure to do the job alone, so radiation was also in the cards. From what I had read thus far, proceeding directly to external beam radiation treatment with an enlarged gland such as mine held the strong likelihood of even more serious long-term side effects.

In this traditional prostate cancer treatment, a powerful beam is aimed precisely at the point of the cancerous tumor and at intervals over a period of time until the cancer cells are destroyed. Commonly, these treatments cover a period of 5 to 6 weeks and require patients to undergo treatment five times per week.

Most urologic surgeons report that one of their major tasks is to eventually correct the postoperative effects of radiation therapy, since there is a fairly high incidence of incontinence, impotence, or both. Clinical evidence also shows that when applied to prostate cancers of low volume and early stage, external beam radiation yields reasonably good results.

At the moment, these were the only options I knew. What course of treatment had the best chance of first stopping cancer growth and then ultimately destroying the cancer?

In *Head First,* Norman Cousins wrote: "In general, anything that restores a sense of control to a patient can be a profound aid to the physician in treating serious illness. That sense of control is more than a mere mood or attitude, and may well be a vital pathway between the brain, the endocrine system, and the immune system. The assumed possibility is that it may serve as the basis for what may well be a profound advance in the knowledge of how to comfort the challenge of a serious illness."

Slowly and carefully, Dr. Wehle now proposed a strategy for treatment that provided us with a series of choices. The first truth to learn is that any treatment of prostate cancer carries with it the side effect of destroying part of your body. As a side effect, you come to accept that a part of yourself is transformed in the process. A new person emerges from the battle. It is a bit like coming home from a war, wounded but unbowed. Prostate cancer bestows upon the male patient the civilian version of the Purple Heart.

Norman Cousins noted: "The way the doctor delivers a diagnosis; the way he creates an environment conducive to effective medical treatment; the way he inspires a patient to become a full partner in a strategy for recovery; the way he takes into account the emotional needs both of the patient and members of the family—all these factors are involved in an effective patient-physician relationship. The major advances in modern medical science give substance to the principle that the mind of the patient creates the ambiance of treatment. Belief becomes the biology. The head comes first."

An Investigational Alternative

Next, Dr. Wehle carefully introduced the subject of cryosurgery (also called cryotherapy), a treatment alternative that was totally unfamiliar to us. Technically, the procedure is called cryoablation of the prostate (*cryo*, "cold"; *ablation*, "removal or destruction of a part of the body"). Cryosurgery, when properly administered, results in total removal of the prostate, as does the radical prostatectomy procedure. He cautioned that cryosurgery was still considered an *investigational procedure*, which is a technical classification by the federal Food and Drug Administration (FDA) during the evaluative stages of approval. The equipment used, however, already carried FDA approval.

The "investigational" designation for cryosurgery immediately raised the question of insurance reimbursement. At the time, most insurance carriers were reluctant to reimburse for this procedure, and it was unclear whether my carrier would cover it. Right up front the doctor raised this warning for my consideration.

Shortly after giving serious thought to cryosurgery, I quickly pulled together the information on my particular case and the available literature on the growing experience with cryosurgery at other institutions. I phoned my group insurance carrier and reviewed my preliminary findings. Next, I was asked to formulate an inquiry letter that outlined the background of my case. Finally, the doctor formalized this process with an official letter request, supported by technical data related to my case and the proposed course of treatment. This three-step process proved successful, and reimbursement was confirmed by my carrier.

The Mayo Clinic Jacksonville had decided to introduce cryosurgery for selected cases and was soon expecting delivery of the necessary equipment. My case seemed to fit the criteria. Successful treatment of a stage T3 prostate cancer with aggressive cell growth "fell between the cracks" of traditional treatments.

Cryosurgery is a procedure of destroying cancerous cells in the prostate gland through freezing it with liquid nitrogen at a temperature $-196°$ C. A transrectal ultrasound machine is used to guide the placement of probes and to monitor the freezing process. The abnormal tissue destroyed by the extreme cold is left in place and is sloughed off or reabsorbed by the body.

Cryosurgical techniques have been under investigation for more than two decades. But only recently—with the advent of new equipment that makes it possible to see exactly where to guide the probe and with the use of liquid nitrogen, which is more temperature controllable than nitrogen gas—could urologic surgeons gain sufficient control of the "freezing zone" to use it in treating large numbers of prostate cancer cases.

At the time of my introduction to this alternative, fewer than 1000 prostate cancer patients had been treated with cryosurgery nationally. More than half of the cases had been treated at Allegheny General Hospital in Pittsburgh, where Dr. Jeffrey Cohen led the urologic team that had refined the techniques and the equipment.

There were no recent 5- and 10-year clinical reports to support the effectiveness of cryosurgery of the prostate. At this point that seemed an interesting but rather academic matter, since I needed to choose a course of action *now*. Otherwise, I stood absolutely no chance of eventually learning of long-term study results.

If cryosurgery were to be my window on life, my procedure would be scheduled for about 3 months from then, when the equipment was scheduled to arrive at the Mayo Clinic. As one of the lead doctors from Pittsburgh, Dr. Cohen would perform the procedure and personally train the Mayo Clinic surgeons and staff in administering the procedure. If this were going to be in the cards for me, there remained a few intermediate hurdles to get over.

First, it would be necessary to *debulk* (reduce) the size of my prostate gland from its present enlarged state. The debulking of the prostate is intended to increase the margin areas within which the surgeons must eventually do their work. Cryosurgery required a maximum-sized target of 45 grams, or about 20% smaller than the size of my prostate gland at that point. This would be accomplished by administering a combination hormone treatment once monthly to stop the production of testosterone, the culprit that was feeding the fast-growing cancer cells.

Next, it was necessary to find out whether the cancer had spread to the lymph nodes adjacent to the prostate. With a 50-50 chance that the cancer had already spread, this procedure became a threshold event. One study concluded that in cases such as mine, with both a high PSA and poorly differentiated cell growth, the odds of cancer having already spread to the lymph nodes were better than 90%. If the cancer was found to have spread, surgery of any kind was out of the question.

As described earlier, in a radical prostatectomy, if the cancer has been found to have spread beyond the prostate gland to the adjacent lymph glands during the radical procedure, it is unwarranted to proceed with removal of the prostate. The same holds true for cryosurgery, except in this case, it requires a separate procedure to determine the condition of the lymph nodes. There had to be an "all clear" sounded and no sign of any spreading for me to qualify for the main event—cryosurgery.

This meant scheduling an exploratory procedure, a laparoscopic lymph node dissection, in which the surgeon makes small incisions through the abdomen to withdraw samples of the seminal vesicles and check the lymph nodes for any signs of malignancy.

My mind flashed back to film director Elia Kazan's classic movie, *On the Waterfront,* in which Marlon Brando plays a former prizefighter who, as a truculent laborer on the New York docks, cries, "You don't understand!" to his brother. "I could have had class. I could have been a contender! I could have been *somebody,* instead of a bum, which is what I am." I felt the same way about my getting my title shot with cryosurgery. Brando's character continues, "He gets a title shot outdoors in a ballpark and I get a one-way ticket to palooka-ville." I too knew that I had to first make it in the "preliminary bout" before being invited to climb into the ring for the main event.

Hormonal treatment and cryosurgery presented an innovative but tortuous dilemma, causing me to want to ponder for a short while. Cynthia, on the other hand, was ready to go for it on the spot. It did seem to offer a new best option under these difficult and dangerous circumstances. We left, drove around the block, and talked about it for a few minutes. We returned shortly.

♦ **Taking Charge Advisory 9:** Move your case if that is warranted.

Second Opinions

Second opinions are a valuable medical tool, too infrequently used in many instances, and overused in others. Clearly, you do not want to get another physician's opinion on every ailment or problem, but in the following situations you should definitely seek out a second opinion:

- Before major surgery
- When the diagnosis is serious or life threatening
- If a rare disease has been diagnosed
- If the diagnosis is uncertain
- If the treatment suggested is risky or expensive
- If the number of tests or procedures seems excessive
- If you are uncomfortable with the diagnosis or treatment
- If a course of treatment is not working
- If you question the competence, thoroughness, or commitment of your doctor
- If your insurance company requires it

Most doctors are supportive of obtaining a second opinion, and many will recommend it. In many cases, insurance companies will pay for second opinions, but you should check ahead of time to make certain your insurance plan covers it. Even if they do not cover it, don't let that discourage you from taking this important step.

Often the opinion of a second doctor affirms the opinion of the first, but the reassurance proves to be worth the time and extra cost. On the other hand, if the second opinion differs markedly from the first, you have two remaining alternatives. You can seek the opinion of a third doctor or you can educate yourself as much as possible by talking with both doctors and reading up on the problems and then trusting your instincts about which diagnosis and course of treatments are correct for you.

If the diagnosis is the same but the recommended treatments differ, as was the situation with my stage T3 prostate cancer, it is important to remember that doctors may have different solutions to the same problem—and both could work. One might work better than the other, or they could both work equally well. However, it is important to remember that *surgical solutions can rarely be reversed.*

The choice was to be based on my preference after considerable research into the subject. It is also advisable to listen closely to what a doctor says about a second opinion. Both in my situation and with my friend Lou Steflik, our physicians had sounded an alarm about the wisdom of obtaining a second opinion from the Mayo Clinic. The first time I heard this, it raised a red flag in my mind. The second time, it caused the flag to flap briskly. From an economic perspective, the practice of medicine is viewed as a cost-centered business venture. For the customer, it remains to be seen whether it is also a *patient-focused* healing enterprise.

Risk and Reward—No Guarantees

One thing must be said about Dr. Wehle—he calls it as he sees it. In his words, he would rather "hang black crepe" than oversell an approach. On the positive side, cryosurgery seemed to offer many of the promises that a radical prostatectomy, radiation therapy, or both combined could not offer to *my statistical case of one.* There was an impressive number of technical papers and case studies that I eventually devoured and digested. On the down side, only a short track record supported the efficacy of the procedure. Thus far, most cryosurgery cases had been performed on stage T1 and T2 cases. Only a few had been stage T3. Nonetheless, results to date seemed promising.

The first positive treatment action was to receive a combination of flutamide (Eulexin) and leuprolide acetate (Lupron Depot) shots (see the Glossary). This began the process of changing my hormonal balance by immediately slowing and eventually shutting down both prostate and adrenal gland production of testosterone.

It seems chance *does* favor the prepared mind. To me, the two-pronged approach made immediate sense; stop feeding the cancer while shrinking the gland, then determine the status of the disease.

Cryosurgery was a new and hopeful possibility. There were positive actions to be taken now; there was more to be learned later. There were new options to be managed. And the physician member of my new team immediately engendered trust.

- He had considerable experience treating this disease.
- He was open to new forms of treatment.
- He involved us in the decision process from the outset.
- He paid close attention to our questions; he gave no "stock" answers.
- He seemed to *care for me as a person,* and for us as a family.

♦ **Taking Charge Advisory 10:** Expand your information base.

Cancer cells thrive on testosterone. To produce testosterone, the body needs to produce a naturally occurring substance called luteinizing hormone–releasing hormone (LH-RH). To halt production of testosterone from the testes, a synthetic substance similar to LH-RH, leuprolide, is injected monthly. Flutamide is an antiandrogen substance that can counteract the biologic effects of the hormones in body cells that depend on androgens. Flutamide works at the site of hormonally dependent prostate cancer cells by preventing the adrenal androgens from being used as a source for nourishing them. Therefore the cancer cells are immediately attacked at two levels: at the testes, using leuprolide, and at the adrenal glands, using flutamide.

A call to Allegheny General Hospital in Pittsburgh produced a next-day package with an abundance of information and reports of clinical studies on cryosurgery. It was vital for me to see all of the available clinical evidence, both good and bad, related to this investigative course of treatment.

Opportunity Knocks

I have carried the following quotation in my wallet for many years. On occasion, a copy has gone to one of my kids or to a friend who has asked for it. At no time in my life did its advice carry greater meaning.

Johann Wolfgang von Goethe wrote: "The moment one definitely commits oneself, then providence moves too. All sorts of things occur to help one that would never otherwise have occurred. A whole stream of events issues from the decision, raising in one's favor all manner of unforeseen incidents and meetings and material assistance which no man could have dreamed would have come his way. Whatever you can do or dream you can, begin it. Boldness has genius, power and magic in it. Begin it now."

Later in the week I met with a business associate who knew of my situation and who was interested to learn of my progress. Some men are very private about these matters, choosing to keep things to themselves. Take the husband of one of my recent graduate students as an example. My student, a middle-aged black woman, came to me and confided that she would be unable to attend the last class for the final examination in Current Economic Analysis. After careful questioning I learned that her husband had just been diagnosed with prostate cancer. An "ex-football player and macho jock," in her words, he refused to talk to anyone, including her, about what the doctors had found. He just accepted the fact that this was it; he was going to die young (age 55), and that was that. I shared an early draft of this book with her to help her bridge the gap, to learn how to deal with the issues. His was a low-grade prostate cancer. He eventually opened up and later she called to tell me that his surgery had turned out well. She also "aced" the final.

My view of sharing information is to be open about it. While not relishing the idea of talking about my illness, I decided early on that it could prove invaluable to share with others a tactful amount of what was going on in my life. An opportunity to do just that almost immediately presented itself.

By providence (or Goethe), one of my clients told me about his father who had undergone cryosurgery for prostate cancer in Pittsburgh about 6 months earlier with Dr. Jeffrey Cohen. The patient, a prominent Florida executive, was a very private man. We talked by phone a few days later. The conversation proved reassuring. I picked up first-hand knowledge about cryosurgery from someone who just 6 months earlier had been where I was considering going. I learned about the intricacies of the procedure, potential postoperative problems, and his healing results, which seemed to be progressing more slowly than expected, from the *patient's* point of view. Next, we compared notes on the similarities as well as the differences in our respective cases: PSA levels, Gleason scores, cell type, prostate size, and so on. (This is where knowing the facts of your own case can be priceless.) He also introduced me to Patient Advocates for Advanced Cancer Treatments, Inc. (PAACT), which acts as a clearinghouse for prostate cancer treatment information as well as a patient advocate group and lobbies for legislation to promote prostate cancer education and research.

One call to PAACT and I was flooded with sets of technical papers, accompanied by dozens of case studies and testimonials from prostate cancer patients across the country. PAACT furnishes relevant and timely information to prostate cancer patients and physicians without cost or obligation, depending solely on contributions to keep their fine work going. The data were to prove vital quite soon thereafter. However, when reviewing any new information base accompanied by strong opinions, the reader must place the source and their conclusions in the proper context. Always keep in mind the origin of the input.

Notwithstanding this caution, you should contact PAACT, US TOO! International, Inc., the American Foundation for Urologic Disease (A.F.U.D.), and others if you face the dilemmas of prostate cancer (see Chapter 9 and Appendix D).

Teamwork Pays Off

Gradually I began to sense that I was "getting my arms around this monster" and allowed myself to feel a bit more confident. For the first time since diagnosis, we were doing something about treating this dread disease. Also, within hours, I could feel the flutamide capsules and leuprolide injections beginning to do their work. Each day I would visualize the prostate gland being starved and getting smaller.

With each passing day I felt that I was beginning to better understand my case. Treatment options were thoroughly discussed with the doctor and family members. We could objectively deal with the pros and cons of alternative courses of action. The time was approaching when these findings, opinions, and a proposed course of action would be put to the test. I talked in great detail with Cynthia, my sons, and other family members about these and other findings to make sure I had not overlooked some small aspect. We debated the risks as well as the benefits of different approaches to my case, especially the wisdom of proceeding with an investigational treatment. My sons continued to hit me with the hard-to-answer questions— subjects that forced me to address complex challenges. The boys also knew what was at stake. They were not going to let me get off easy— and that was great.

About this time the current issue of *Scientific American* featured an article entitled "The Dilemma of Prostate Cancer Treatment." Great timing! Goethe again?

Living with prostate cancer and its yet-undetermined postoperative effect promised to be difficult for me as well as for those who care for me. Everyone involved faced a host of problems, challenges, and choices. Decisions would soon have to be made at a fast and furious tempo.

Cynthia attended several American Cancer Society Man to Man support group meetings and met other wives of prostate cancer patients. The most often repeated questions dealt with the options available if the husband becomes incontinent, impotent, or both. Although the man is the cancer victim, the woman and the family are increasingly affected.

In general, women are more concerned about health issues than are men, and women are often more comfortable talking about these issues. By sharing information about prostate cancer, a woman may save a man a great deal of difficulty and possibly even his life (see Chapter 10).

Cynthia planned a simple, nourishing diet for me with more emphasis than before on fresh vegetables and fruits. My wife is a very determined woman and a real scrapper. Little by little she took responsibility for superintending my diet, caring for the house with less and less help from me, and rearranging our life to meet the new challenges—all of this while holding down a full-time job that she did not particularly like. She made certain that our evenings and weekends included taking a little extra time to smell the roses, to travel to the beach a mile from our home to watch the surf rolling in and out. We kept up our daily exercise schedule, regardless of how debilitated I might feel as a result of my medications. There was no letup in my daily dose of vitamins either. As the countdown continued toward my surgery, Cynthia stepped up my exercise schedule. You have to be strong and in shape before undergoing the rigors of surgery.

Each evening meal would begin with a toast, *L'Hiam*, the Yiddish expression that means "to life," made popular by the song of the same name in the Broadway show and movie *Fiddler on the Roof*. To this day, our children and grandchildren begin each family meal together, even at McDonalds, by clinking together their glasses, or Styrofoam cups, and wishing one another *L'Hiam*. Not once in all this time did I ever hear Cynthia complain. At the outset we prioritized our project objectives together. It brought us even closer than either of us could have imagined. These goals were to (1) destroy the cancer and get out of this with my life; (2) try to avoid or heal incontinence; and (3) reinvigorate and *reinvent* our sex lives as healing progressed.

There can be no greater support group leader than your wife backed by family members and other loved ones. At times like this a lifetime of love bears fruit. Busy business guys ought to keep in mind that "no one ever lies on his deathbed wishing he had spent more time at the office."

Chapter 6

Nine Underlying Principles

♦ **Taking Charge Advisory 11:** Keep updating the project schedule.

The tempo of change caused us to continually readjust our timetable. First, the presurgical program now called for enough time to allow combination hormone treatment to start working. The expected
result was to block the cancer growth by shutting down the production of testosterone in both the prostate and the adrenal glands and to
debulk the size of the prostate, which would take about 3 months. But
how would we know if it was working?

Men are familiar with the process of hormonal change that takes
place in women during middle age. Telltale hot flashes reveal this
process of change in a woman's body chemistry. The same is true for
a man. Therapeutic hormone treatments affect a man the same way.

Are the Hot Flashes Worth It?

Within just a few days of the first leuprolide injection, my hot
flashes came on and continued for about a year after injections were
stopped. Almost hourly a wave of heat and sweat came over me. Hot
flashes are usually short lived, often lasting only minutes, and can be
precipitated by environmental changes such as getting into a hot car
on a spring day. During the night, Cynthia and I would wake up and
start laughing. Is that you or me? It was nice to have someone going
through it with me, so there was understanding. That, of course, is
what she said also.

My middle son Ken was trained as an architect and is a very prac-
tical guy. After watching me break into a hot flash episode, he hit on
a capital idea. Ken brought me a small handheld battery-operated fan

from a discount store. At the first rise in body temperature, I pointed the fan toward my neck and, low and behold, the breeze broke the heat cycle, allowing me to cool down more quickly. It was an imaginative solution to an annoying problem—I was well equipped for battle.

We knew the hormone treatments were hard at work. With each episode I visualized the hot flash as depriving the cancer cells of nourishment. It was gratifying to *feel* those results every hour. This was serious business. Viewed as an indicator of effectiveness, hot flashes became a downright exhilarating event.

As soon as the prostate cancer patient begins the combination hormone therapy, the disease is being treated. As a result, tumor growth is halted, the prostate gland begins to shrink, and thus in most cases the PSA level also begins to drop.

After 10 days of combination therapy and 3 months of leuprolide injections, my prostate volume decreased by about 25%. This brought the size of the gland well within the acceptable target range for cryosurgery. My PSA level also fell from its previous 41.8 down to 1.

At this point, the results were so good I was ready to declare victory. However, this combination hormone therapy is not prescribed as the sole long-term treatment because eventually cancer cells, if not destroyed by some other means, begin to feed on the synthetic hormone and cancer growth resumes. One member of a support group reported that his PSA began to rise again after being on hormone treatment for more than 5 years.

The First Cliffhanger

If the PSA level is 20.0 or higher, there is considerable concern that the cancer may have already spread to the adjacent lymph nodes. Thus, as I discussed earlier, it is prudent for the urologist to examine the lymph nodes to determine to what extent, if any, there has been a spread of prostate cancer. As I have said, my doctor estimated that there was a more than 50-50 chance the cancer had already spread at this stage. However, one clinical study reported that with a PSA level as elevated as mine, there was a 95% chance that it had already spread. I assured my sister Shirley that I could do more with a 5% chance than most people can do with 95%. Sure, I was scared, but I had to maintain a positive mind-set.

Approximately 50% of the body's pelvic lymph nodes can be examined by means of laparoscopic surgery. An exploratory examination is performed with a laparoscopic lymph node dissection procedure. In this method, the surgeon views the organs within the abdomen through a scope mounted on a slender instrument that has a self-contained camera unit. The surgeon also withdraws samples of lymph nodes located close to the prostate for examination under a microscope in the pathology laboratory.

I underwent a laparoscopic lymph node dissection in April, 3½ months after my initial diagnosis. The doctor sought out Cynthia in the waiting room. She had been valiantly struggling to concentrate on reading *Truman*, a biography. It had been about 7 hours since she had kissed me and wished me well as I rolled into the operating room. The doctor took her to a small one-on-one-sized room, where he told her that the pathology laboratory had sent word that the lymph nodes were clear and that the cancer had not spread farther. In a daze, she walked back across the crowded surgical waiting room and, as she approached her chair, grabbed the armrest; her legs had turned to rubber and given out. She broke down and sobbed. Word was waiting for me when I came out from under anesthesia. The lymph nodes were clear; the cancer had not spread. I had made the finals!

On reflection, even as I review these words, it does not now seem possible to describe our feeling of exhilaration. Joy was mixed with great relief. It was truly another *celebrative experience*, such as when you have overcome great odds—the underdog winning the big game.

In *Man's Search for Meaning*, Victor Frankl describes his prolonged experience as a prisoner in a Nazi concentration camp: "There are three main avenues on which one arrives at the meaning of life. The first is by creating work or by doing a deed. The second is by experiencing something or encountering someone; in other words, meaning can be found not only in work but also in love. Most important, however, is the third avenue to meaning in life: facing a fate he cannot change, may rise above himself, may grow beyond himself, and by so doing change himself. He may turn a personal tragedy into a triumph."

Patients on their way to treatment centers are usually in a state of fear—fear of procedures that are unfamiliar and often threatening, fear of the equipment used, fear of disease, and general fear of the unknown. The goal of the health provider (physician, nurse, PA, technician, support person) needs to be to humanize the environment and to help reduce the stress of undergoing medical procedures. Why?

- The body is more robust than most people had previously believed. Its ability to bounce back from illness tells us that treatments, especially with medications, should be tempered—and this knowledge needs to be part of every American's health education.
- A patient may quickly panic. The physician's skill in reassuring the patient can be a significant factor in stimulating the body's natural healing process; it can help magnify treatment.
- The astute physician always gives careful attention to the many conditions that surround health care; it can affect the result.
- Positive emotions such as the will to live, love, tenacity, resolve, and humor actually produce biochemical responses that can affect the outcome of medical care.
- Depression has been found to be a cause of physical illness, including damage to the immune system.
- Although a positive patient attitude is not a guarantee of a cure, it can help both the patient and physician to get the most out of health care.
- Patients tend to move along the path of their expectations, both up and down.
- Since unexpected remissions do occur (many have been reported in medical journals), both physicians and patients are justified in hoping for and working for the best.
- In treatment, a good challenge beats a grim verdict. The patient must make a special effort and believe the effort is worthwhile.
- Emotional shattering often follows a serious diagnosis. Family, friends, and support groups can all help offset the fear of being alone.
- Medical technology does not replace a physician's diagnostic skills. The patient's mind-set when taking diagnostic tests can affect the test outcome.
- The physician's ability to listen to and hear the patient is as important as medical test printouts. Understanding the factors that preceded the illness is as important as identifying the pathologic process.

The majority of people I have encountered in health care—nurses, doctors, professional assistants, secretaries, administrators—can hold their heads high in terms of work quality, high purpose, and an insightful understanding of their profession.

Getting Ready for the Main Event

At this point there were two tasks. First, I had to prepare myself and my family in the event things did not work out as planned. Second, I had to forge ahead for a positive result. These tasks may not be as mutually exclusive as you might think.

On the first score it meant cleaning up my debts, taking care to get all of my papers in order, committing to telling my family and friends that I loved them as often as possible, spending time with myself reflecting on my life's accomplishments, spending time fortifying my inner being, leaving a few moments to cry together with my wife, making certain to enjoy myself a little more, and making peace with myself—this meant acceptance of what is.

On moving ahead vigorously with decisive action to knock out the cancer, I did all of the above as well as stepping up my last-minute information search. Three months earlier I had walked into the Mayo Clinic with scant knowledge about prostate cancer diagnosis, treatment, and healing. Now I had learned a great deal about cryosurgery, its potential benefits as well as its limitations.

My search also included turning to the Internet, the worldwide information network, which at the time was technically still quite primitive. This was before the coming of today's sophisticated Web browser. We accessed sites using an extension of e-mail. I searched for sources of prostate cancer research, the National Institutes of Health and the National Cancer Institute. It included downloading reports, phoning for copies of studies, and reading statistical tables (see Appendix D).

The same studies were repeatedly read and reread. I needed to be certain that I fully understood what they were saying. They were not written for lay persons, and they had a language all their own (see the Glossary). More important was that I grasp what all of the data, discussion, and conclusions meant in relation to *my specific case.*

A significant number of clinical trials take place in many parts of

the world. Clinical trials seek to evaluate the effectiveness of new research treatments. The National Cancer Institute was contacted by e-mail and response came from the Cancer Information Service. PAACT was very supportive and never stopped the deluge of timely materials on patient experiences, patient options, and cryosurgery facts and opinions. They strongly endorsed cryosurgery but in fact may be overselling its applicability for all patients. The personnel at Allegheny General Hospital in Pittsburgh remained genuinely cooperative.

At the time, I was unaware of US TOO! International, Inc., which has now organized more than 500 prostate cancer support groups worldwide, or the American Foundation for Urologic Disease (A.F.U.D.), with more than 450 affiliated support groups. Both have been commended by and are evaluated by an American Urological Association (AUA) board of advisors. A.F.U.D. is in the forefront of many worthwhile efforts related to prostate cancer. The A.F.U.D. Research Scholar Program was developed 20 years ago by the AUA to encourage outstanding investigators in urologic research. Since 1987, this program has allocated more than $14 million to 300 investigators, more than 90% of whom have continued their careers in urologic research. In 1996 A.F.U.D. distributed $3 million to 81 researchers. Approximately one third of this research will focus on prostate cancer and other prostate diseases. US TOO! International, Inc. also offers one-on-one support services with knowledgeable prostate cancer survivors (see Appendix D).

We studied success stories as well as failures. Protocol studies on patients following failure of radical prostatectomy procedures were especially illuminating. Genetic research programs were made available. Postprocedure results for external beam radiation and cryosurgery were calculated. I even came across the story of a prostate cancer patient who tried to shoot his urologist (fortunately, he missed) when the patient realized "the feeling of making love will never be part of my life again." Patient testimonials detailing their outcomes with cryosurgery were forwarded to us. There was no shortage of studies, but no clear consensus of approach or results.

The fall 1994 issue of *Cancer Communication*, published by PAACT, summarized a study conducted by A.F.U.D. and the Gallup Organization. It included the following answers to the question, "Where do prostate cancer patients obtain information?" The findings were as follows (some patients reported gathering information from several sources):

- Doctors, 43%
- Support groups, 32%
- Cancer organizations, 30%
- Magazines, 16%
- Newspapers, 9%
- Library, 9%

- Family, 2%
- Universities, 6%
- Don't know, 1%
- Cancer hotline, <0.5%
- Other, 4%

Calculating the Odds

The more studies I read, prostate survivors I talked with, books, newspapers, and magazine articles I reviewed, television reports I watched, and the more I reflected on the subject, the more I was convinced that *each case is a statistical case of one.*

You can find almost any answer you want in the reports. No single report I read contained completely relevant information when compared with *my* particular set of prostate screening data. The more I tried to piece together different findings, the more apparent it became that *the parts came from different puzzles.* Therefore those parts did not fit together so neatly when I was trying to reach a conclusion.

There are many bad jokes about statistics. For example, "Statistics means never having to say you're certain." One saying has stayed with me since my teen years as a Red Cross lifeguard: "A 6-foot man can just as easily drown in an average of 3 feet of water." It was urgent that I learn to swim in all this information!

♦ **Taking Charge Advisory 12:** Understand that yours is a statistical case of one.

It may be useful to again remind readers that the approaches I selected and used in the treatment and healing of my particular case of prostate cancer are in no way suggested to be the right answer for your situation, nor would I expect the outcome to be the same for your particular case.

The Medical Team

The idea of a patient-physician partnership is not just an admirable theory but a genuine functional necessity.

As events are presently unfolding in the health provider field (physician groups, hospitals, HMOs, insurance carriers, Medicare, and Medicaid), Norman Cousins' words reverberate with new meaning: "Few things are more essential for the national future than the need for Americans to be reeducated about health: education about internal and external mechanisms for warding off disease or coping with it, should it occur; education in the requirements of good health; education that can teach us that panic and defeat are the great multipliers of illness; education about the importance of confidence in repair, restoration, recovery, regeneration; education in the need for a partnership between patient and physician; education in what is meant by the human healing system and how it works best; education in the value of putting our best effort toward maximizing what is possible; and finally, education that can instruct us that what goes on in the mind can promote or restore health."

The time was growing near when all that I had learned over the past few months would be used to help decide the course of action for destroying the cancer in my body. Right or wrong, here is how I finally sized up *my* statistical case of one:

- My stage T3 cancer could not be completely removed by radical prostatectomy; some residual cancer would remain, meaning a full series of radiation treatments to follow.
- Because of the enlarged size of my prostate, the margins available for radical prostatectomy were less than adequate. There would be a great risk of damaging the sphincter area (the muscles that control continence) from surgery and radiation.
- Residual branching of remaining cancer cells not reached by the scalpel might tend to accelerate their spread to other parts of the body.
- External beam radiation treatment on such a large gland could most likely cause other damage while concentrating its effectiveness at the prostate and bladder areas.
- Cryosurgery, as I saw it, had a good potential for removing cancer from the entire area. It works like a *heat sink,* attracting the

heat of the cancer cells *to* the ice ball created by the freezing process, since cancer cells are *hotter* than normal cells and are attracted first. One stray cell could eventually kill me.

- The heat sink principle is what happens when you get out of a warm swimming pool and feel cold. The cooler air draws heat quickly *from* your warm body.
- Liquid nitrogen can be effectively controlled. The cryosurgical probe, placed through the perineum into the prostate gland, forms an ice ball. This draws heat not only from within the gland but from all areas defined as the margin.
- The best chance of killing any stray cancer cells and keeping them from getting away was to draw them to the ice ball.
- The postoperative effects of cryosurgery held the promise of being less debilitating over the long term than a radical prostatectomy because of the less invasive nature of the procedure.

This summed up the *pluses* about it, the *minuses* about it, and what was *interesting* about it—the PMI. Cryoablation of the prostate seemed to add up to me as the most promising alternative course of treatment in my situation.

The How and Why of Finding Solutions

Project management is built on reasoning, problem solving, and decision making. When you use intuition, you make an overall or global evaluation of how you *feel* about a course of action. When researchers compare the intuitive judgments of people (including experts) to a standard, intuitive decision makers invariably do poorly because the more complex the system that we are dealing with (and prostate cancer falls in that category), the more counterintuitive seems to be the result of purely intuitive decision making. For more than 30 years, the System Dynamics program at the Massachusetts Institute of Technology has devoted considerable effort to demonstrating why unintended consequences occur.

Effectively managing the decisions related to the treatment and healing of prostate cancer, a life-threatening disease, calls for a clear vision of the necessary activities. Situations arise without warning, calling for quick and sure response. It calls for strengthening both the rational and the intuitive aspects in the decision process. These responses can be summarized into a framework of nine underlying principles.

Nine Underlying Priniciples
for Decision Making and Problem Solving

1. Successful people question both *how* and *why* they must spend time and effort to find solutions. This is the basic principle that gives us the key to power. It is an efficient and effective tool for determining how to approach the problem, why you want or need to solve it, and your satisfaction with potential solutions.

2. Every problem exists as a class of one. It is unique because it lies in a framework unlike any other; it is contextually unique. The further we explore the potential result of different treatments, the more this principle takes shape.

3. Every problem must be addressed *polyperceptually,* that is, we must deliberately think about a problem and act on a solution after gathering information from various points of view. No single clinical study or professional opinion should suffice in tackling and solving such a complex problem.

4. We must be sure that we are working on the *right problem.* Problems have many disguises and aliases. We can only be sure if we explore the meaning of the problem to us and our purposes for exerting time and effort to find solutions. In my case the trade-off between short-term and long-term results was consistently tested.

5. We must try to find what we perceive to be an ideal solution. Breakthroughs in thinking are always strengthened by our working back from some ideal solution. Understanding our priorities helped set the parameters for selecting the most appropriate treatment option.

6. Every problem is part of a *technically defined mess.* It is always embedded in and interconnected with other problems. It is part of some system. At first it is easy to get caught up in the prevailing wisdom and lose sight of its applicability to the specific case.

7. Seeking other points of view is a *cooperative activity.* We must approach it through cooperative competition—seeking believers and doubters. Literature searches, hearing other patients' experiences, and seeking a second opinion set the stage for challenging the original decision.

8. It is possible to suffer *mental indigestion,* or data overload. We must avoid "knowing too much." In its place we must learn how to *structure the information* so it helps us to make an informed decision.

9. Life, like love and liberty, must be won anew; we must regenerate our lifeforce. The task is not to build up a complicated mix of factors, but rather to *reduce* a large number of initial possibilities to one—the appropriate course of action.

♦ **Taking Charge Advisory 13:** Build a positive mind-set.

The Positive Mind-Set

Warren, my youngest son, is a professional photographer in New York. Several years ago I gave him a copy of *I Ching*, the ancient Chinese source book. In my present plight he sent me a copy of Joyce Sequichie Hifler's *A Cherokee Feast of Days* (Council Oak Publishing, Tulsa, Oklahoma, 1992). Each morning, the Cherokee Indian meditations for that day proved inspirational and timely. Let me share with you the readings for two eventful days.

On April 20, before I headed to the hospital for the laparoscopic lymph node dissection, the cliffhanging qualifying round, I read:

An idea is a rare butterfly that leads us through visual and spiritual experiences, and brings us out of the woods changed and ready to do something we never dreamed possible. Most people catch hold of ideas and immediately say they take too much time and money to be worth the effort. A quick excuse has cut more people out of doing a profitable and rewarding deed than all other work put together. Fear of failure chips away at self-confidence until there is no heart to step into new territory. One needs the mind of a child to forget what happened an hour ago. If we cannot forget, we put it aside until we get to a place where we can understand; otherwise, our creativity knows no bounds. We are caught up in a world of imagination—the thing that blesses all great inventors—playing what-if and finding great treasure.*

On May 4, before my date with the cryosurgery probes, I read:

Little things speak to our hurts. Sounds, fragrances, music that would mean nothing to others, reach into our souls to do work that the obvious could not touch. Simple remedies can heal the deepest ills—a smile, a contented whistle of a passerby, the sound of birds twittering at dusk—these things warm us and give us hope. But we have to listen for voices, inner and outer, to give us rest—and turn away the negative talk, the negative circumstance. We don't always believe we have a choice—but we have more space to work there than we know. We can no longer scoff at the power to help our-

---

*Reprinted with permission of Council Oak Publishing from *A Cherokee Feast of Days* by Joyce Sequichie Hifler, copyright © 1992 by Joyce Hifler.

selves. We have a bigger hand in it than imagined, and it is our decision to get down to business and be open to help and healing from unlikely sources.*

My daughter Erica gave me a copy of Dr. Bernie Siegel's *Love, Medicine & Miracles*. The book is rich with patient stories and leaves the reader with a sense of renewed hope.

The world of the operating room, when viewed from the table, takes on a terrifying prospect. A patient looks up at big bright lights, uniforms, and masks. If this is the last thing the patient sees before the black rubber mouthpiece goes on, this is not a satisfying or sustaining image for the subconscious to carry through surgery. But when the patient knows that his teammate, his own doctor, is near him and can feel a compassionate hand on his shoulder, his apprehensions are eased and his confidence nourished.

The day before cryosurgery I met with PA Ryan and Dr. Wehle to go over some last-minute details and home preparation. I was to drink a quart of something innocently called GoLytely laced with lemon-flavored Crystal Light. GoLytely is a bowel-cleansing preparation routinely administered before surgical procedures near the bowel. This stuff is memorable—its effects are unpleasant, but necessary.

We would all next meet in the operating room in the morning. By now the process was all fairly straightforward. We had come to this point as a team; now, we were ready for the main event. At the last moment, I stood in the doorway, turned to Mike Wehle, extended my hand to his, and said, "Let's go get it!"

♦ **Taking Charge Advisory 14:** Go for it together.

Cryosurgery remains investigational at this writing. As I described earlier, it destroys cancerous cells in the prostate gland by freezing the prostate with liquid nitrogen at −196° C. One clinical report describes the procedure as *annihilating* the prostate. The dead tissue is left in place and is eventually resorbed by the body. The ultimate effect is to remove the prostate through this process.

*Reprinted with permission of Council Oak Publishing from *A Cherokee Feast of Days* by Joyce Sequichie Hifler, copyright © 1992 by Joyce Hifler.

Once the patient is anesthetized, the doctor uses an ultrasound image on a monitor to guide the probe, which is inserted through the perineal area (between the scrotum and rectum) into the prostate. In the prostate, the probe's five needles introduce the full freezing into the gland in a circular, overlapping effect for a specified period of time, as carefully measured by the surgeon. A warming catheter is placed in the urethra to prevent its being damaged by freezing. A suprapubic tube is directly inserted into the bladder, allowing urine to empty into a collection bag. The cryosurgery procedure takes about 2 hours from start to finish.

During that first night my vital signs were routinely taken and recorded, and the next morning the surgical catheter was removed. Karen and Mike (we were now on a first-name basis after all we had been through together) poked their heads in early to check on me. Twenty-four hours later I walked out of the hospital with a tube that came directly from my bladder and was connected to a bag taped onto my leg.

The third morning following "cryo" (we too were now old friends), I went off on my regular walk around the block, although a bit more carefully, with Cynthia and Cookie (my beloved fluffy white mutt). In contrast, the radical prostatectomy had promised to keep me in the hospital for 6 to 8 days! So far, so good.

Chapter 7

Journey to Recovery

Now the Real Work Begins

Up to this point all of my inquiries had turned up information related to the diagnosis and treatment phases of prostate cancer. Little if any mention was made of postoperative care. In part, this probably stems from the fact that each person heals at his own pace. To the physicians' credit, this may also reflect a desire to avoid frightening the patient. They simply want to KISS (keep it simple, stupid) the problem and let events unfold in their own manner and time—and to deal with each postoperative issue as it occurs. Regardless of the rate of healing associated with different treatments and their postoperative effects, it is now the patient's turn to find his own way.

"Some of the things that we read about do not return quite as quickly as advertised," said former Senator Bob Dole, speaking to a *Time* magazine reporter of his healing experience with prostate cancer.

Talking with support group members reveals a surprisingly consistent set of postoperative complications, regardless of the treatment procedure used. Each is more or less severe, depending on the myriad of factors related to *each specific case*. These fall into three main categories:

1. *Pain.* Some postoperative pain in inevitable. Radical prostatectomy patients report considerable pain at the location where the invasive surgery occurs. Radiation leaves behind its own marks of debilitation. Cryosurgery results in a soreness in the perineum, where the cryoprobe was inserted—as though you have ridden a hot motorcycle.

2. *Leakage.* A degree of urinary incontinence seems to come with each of the prostate cancer treatment territories. Often, postoperative scarring complicates return to normal urination. With time, incontinence may heal spontaneously or with Kegel contraction/relaxation exercises, which are designed to strengthen the sphincter muscles. However, minor corrective surgical treatment is sometimes necessary.

3. *Impotence.* It takes time to determine the extent to which potency has been affected by surgery. First, healing must be well on its way. Next, continence needs to be stabilized. Finally, through the period of healing, some experimentation can begin. But it takes several months to more than a year before a final conclusion can be drawn.

Expect Plumbing Problems

Wives or other caregivers must be patient with the man after surgery or radiation treatment. Even if there is no permanent damage to the bladder or nerves, there most likely will be frequent occasions when he will suffer from incontinence (inability to control urination). It is hard enough on the male ego for a man to be performing his voiding chores as if he were an infant; an insensitive wife or caregiver who complains only adds to his distress. A sensitive caregiver is one who talks less, looks more, and devises ways to help the loved one deal with incontinence.

The different types of incontinence are generally classified by the symptoms or circumstances occurring at the time of the leakage. Only much later did I learn that it helps to understand *which* situation you are in so that you can properly discuss it with your physician-partner. At one time or another I went through each stage, although not in any specific order.

A year into my period of the uncertainty of incontinence, we planned a 1-week vacation. I was afraid that the incessant postoperative leakage would ruin our good time, since from time to time my bladder acted as though it had a mind of it own. We had been through some rough times together and needed genuine rest and rehabilitation. Cynthia hit on the idea of my wearing one of those fanny packs, as they are called, to carry extra pads. Then she brought an oversize

Types of Incontinence

- **Stress incontinence** may result from poor bladder support by the pelvic muscles. The condition allows urine leakage when you do anything that strains or stresses the abdomen, such as walking, coughing, sneezing, or laughing.
- **Urge incontinence** results when an overactive bladder contracts without your wanting it to do so. You feel as though you can't wait to reach a toilet. At times you may leak urine with no warning at all. It can be caused by infection or irritation.
- **Mixed incontinence** is often a combination of both of the above conditions—stress and urge incontinence.
- **Overflow incontinence** occurs when the bladder is allowed to become so full that it simply overflows. This happens when bladder weakness or a blocked urethra prevents normal emptying.
- **Environmental incontinence** (sometimes called functional incontinence) occurs when a person cannot get to the toilet when he needs it.
- **Nocturnal enuresis** is incontinence that occurs during sleep.

"shopping bag" type of purse in which she carried an extra change for me if events overtook me. This bolstered my confidence, reduced the stress both of us had felt, and helped to make the trip enjoyable.

My healing was initially pretty slow. For the first month I was unable to void on my own, and the suprapubic tube remained in place as a backup. Frequent bladder spasms also caused me considerable pain. On more than one occasion I called a Mayo Clinic PA who talked me through the steps to reduce the spasm. PA Gary Long helped me through a particularly tough episode at 4 AM one morning. PA Karen Ryan diagnosed over the phone from my reported heavy night sweats that a postoperative bacterial infection had probably set in. After 4 weeks, a severe infection did erupt, requiring an 8-day hospitalization.

It never was clear what had caused this infection or where in the body it was lodged. It was generally believed to lie in the dead prostate tissue. One thing was certain, however. After 30 days, it was absolutely necessary for the doctor to do an exploratory procedure to find out why postoperative voiding was still not normal. General anesthesia was necessary.

Because of the size of my prostate gland at the time of surgery (45 grams, just inside the acceptable range for cryosurgery), a large volume of dead tissue needed to be either absorbed or expelled by the body. That would take some time.

It now looked as though mending was going to progress more slowly and require a longer period than we had originally hoped. Also, it proved vital for me to properly define what was happening so that those frequent telephone talks with a PA, nurse, or the doctor could be productive.

The first question is always whether a patient needs to see a doctor at all. That is the biggest decision the doctor or the PA makes over the phone—talking to the patient, trying to decide whether he is sick enough to need to be seen right now, or whether it can wait. The patient wants to know the same thing. Many patients sometimes spend all night or all weekend trying to reach their doctor, who is off duty, or out of town, or otherwise not immediately available. The issue of accessibility seems to lie with medicine's capacity for dealing with *individuals* rather than groups.

The hospital is also a difficult place to adapt to. A person arrives from the outside and is plunged into new experiences, with new schedules (Does a temperature really need to be taken at 5 AM?), new food (no comment), new clothes (or what there is of a hospital gown to cover a 6-foot, 4-inch frame), new language, new sounds, new smells, new fears, and rewards. For the patient entering this new environment, it seems a foreign place for which there are no guidebooks.

While recovering from infection I must have looked pretty decrepit. My 7-year-old grandson Geoffrey came to visit and asked point-blank, "Are you going to survive, Pop-Pop?" Children have a gift for asking the key question.

A hospital makes psychological demands on the patient that may unintentionally slow recovery. Dependence and loss of power and control are immediately obvious. Inability to tolerate pain and suffering may work at cross purposes with a patient's expectation of getting well.

St. Luke's Hospital in Jacksonville is a Mayo Clinic–affiliated facility with excellent operating standards. I would rate the *caring quotient* of nurses and support staff (how they view and *care for* the patient) as superb.

As my condition improved, I felt less tolerant; I griped more about the food (which my wife insists was not all that bad) and the noises at night (which seemed to reverberate through the body when the nervous system had been jogged). Basically, this patient was becoming less dependent on the surroundings with each day and was increasingly ready to leave. Like most patients, I adjusted well, recovered, and more than happily went home.

Three important benefits resulted from this extended trip to the hospital. First, a cystoscopic examination revealed a blockage of the urethra that could best be repaired on the spot with a small transurethral resection of the prostate (TURP), a procedure commonly used to remove tissue from an enlarged and noncancerous prostate gland—benign prostatic hyperplasia. This incision, which can be pictured like the coring of an apple, removed pressure on the urethra, allowing passage of urine from the bladder so that nature could perform as intended. Second, samples of tissue removed during the TURP procedure were examined by the pathology laboratory under the microscope and found to be free of cancer. With cryosurgery, this was a threshold finding. It is always questionable whether the tissue located closest to the warming catheter, which is used to protect the urethra, could also be effectively frozen and cancer cells destroyed. In this case it worked fine. Third, the infection subsided under heavy bombardment from antibiotics, although it was never clear where it had originated or had been located.

Surgeons have come to see that surgery has the goal of altering the functional status of tissues in the body. This provides the body with the ability to begin to heal itself. But it also calls upon the patient and the body to sacrifice part of itself. The commonly heard expression, "that took a lot out of me," is literally as well as figuratively true of surgery.

With my having completed the exploratory lymph node dissection, cryosurgery, and now the TURP, I had almost completed the *prostate training program*. The doctor cautioned that during the TURP procedure, only a minimal amount of tissue had been removed—enough to do the job. His concern, as always, was that a more extensive procedure might result in permanent damage and incontinence. Possibly, he warned, the procedure might have to be repeated. As described earlier, the finest surgeons are reluctant to operate unless necessary, subscribing to the adage "less is more."

♦ **Taking Charge Advisory 15:** Learn the new tools.

More and more the evidence pointed to what was meant by a statistical case of one. Not that my case was a rarity. Rather, what came through were the indicators that each person's body reacts to treatment in its own unique way. Thus it is all the more important that the patient appreciate what is happening along his path. Cryosurgery was also new to this urologic surgical team and thus the doctor, PAs, nurses, and myself all traveled a new road together. I was Mayo Clinic Jacksonville cryosurgery patient number 2.

None of this suggests that the doctor or any of the staff were unprepared for what was happening or about to happen. On the contrary, I was astonished to watch how quickly this team sensed the significance of each new event. It is a testament to the people skills and standards of these dedicated professionals and to the Mayo Clinic for having found and employed them.

My healing steadily continued, but not uneventfully. Blockages occurred intermittently that required self-catheterization (the insertion of a narrow, lubricated, flexible tube up through the penis and urethra until it enters the bladder). These daily and sometimes 4-times-daily events kept the urethral channel clear and helped remove dead prostate tissue.

One or two naps each day proved to be necessary for some time. Periodically I grabbled for the remote control, flipped on the television, surfed the channels, and turned it off again. I thought of comedian Fred Allen's wisecrack in the early days of television that "TV is a device that permits people who haven't anything to do to watch people who can't do anything." Men have to become acquainted with taking the time to heal. It is not something that comes naturally or easily to us. Dead prostate tissue was gradually being absorbed by my body, but the body ordinarily rejects dead tissue. As a result, sporadic infections developed. The addition of different antibiotics caused continual drowsiness. Over a 12-month period, the sloughing off or discharge of dead tissue into the urethra also caused recurrent episodes of temporary blockage.

Michael Crichton, a physician-turned-novelist, in his first book, *Five Patients*, recounts that during the Civil War surgical mortality from infection was generally 80%. It was during this period that surgeons began to remove dead tissue from wounds to retard infection (debridement). The principle of excising dead tissue as the initial step in wound management finally emerged during World War I.

Some Days Are Better Than Others

In the case of my cryosurgery, the body had to cleanse itself of dead tissue over 12 months. Some things had to be accepted as they unfolded. Soon I could manage my day enough and keep matters under control sufficiently to venture out. It took practice to learn when to call for help and when to ask the health provider team to teach me how to better care for myself.

Information was the critical link in our team's effectiveness. I was brought into the clinic and instructed in the fine art of performing the essential self-treatment steps. I wanted to learn more about why different-sized instruments were prescribed for my home use. On several occasions I discussed directly with the doctor my sense of things and compared notes on the effectiveness of the home treatment, and as a result we agreed that a change in direction was appropriate.

♦ **Taking Charge Advisory 16:** Accept.

Acceptance

Acceptance differs from man to man, from day to day, from hour to hour. What matters, then, is not the meaning of acceptance in general but rather the specific meaning of a person's life at a moment in time. To put the question in general terms would be as though asking a chess champion to tell us, "What is the best chess move in the world?" There is no best move or even an excellent move, apart from a particular situation in a game and the particular personality of one's opponent. The same holds true for understanding acceptance.

Everyone has his specific mission or vocation in life—to carry out an "assignment" that demands fulfillment. As such, he cannot be replaced nor his life be repeated. Everyone's task is unique and is as specific to the individual as his opportunity to implement it, his fingerprints, and his DNA.

The more you forget yourself, by giving yourself to a cause or another person to love, the more human you are and the more you actualize yourself. We find meaning when confronted with a situation that cannot be changed. What is called for, then, is to find ways to turn a personal tragedy into a triumph, to find ways to turn one's predicament into a personal achievement. When we are no longer able to change a situation—such as having and treating T3 prostate cancer, we are challenged to change ourselves.

There are always choices to make. Every day, every hour, offers the opportunity to make a decision—a decision that determines whether you will or will not submit to those events that threaten to rob you of your very self, your inner freedom, that determine whether you will become the victim of circumstance. Bismarck said, "Life is like being at the dentist. You always think the worst is still to come, and yet it is over already."

♦ **Taking Charge Advisory 17:** Progress makes perfect.

Although there were some setbacks, day by day there was progress. I learned to live with them both. Compared to my situation 6 months earlier when all of this first surfaced, I was now traveling the road to recovery. My PSA remained undetectable, tissue samples were negative, and my strength was returning, with only occasional lapses of energy and some temporary blockages. I summed up my feelings to Dr. Wehle.

Dear Dr. Wehle:

I want to take a few moments to share with you my thoughts on the several milestones we have crossed together these past four months.

First, I can't say enough about your excellent care. From the moment Cynthia and I came to you for a second opinion, we immediately felt we had found a physician who would care for my situation as a person and not just a body part. Our initial sense of trust and confidence was tested and borne out under fire several times during these recent months.

Next, the Mayo Clinic health care system is almost indescribable. I know, because I've tried to explain its subtleties to others. Your entire support team has performed first rate. Each PA was very responsive. I probably crossed paths with all of them during this period. Karen Ryan, who has been close to my case from day one, was especially helpful during my ups and downs and patient answering my many questions. Gary Long nursed me through two crises with a smile, even though it meant working through one call at 4:00 in the morning. Your secretary was always pleasant and helpful.

I realize that although the postoperative results have thus far been very encouraging, we are never certain when, or even if, we are ever completely out of the woods. Nonetheless, Cynthia and I feel deeply that your initial diagnosis, recommended treatment strategy, and personal care have given us this renewed lease on life. For that, we will be eternally grateful.

With warmest personal regards,

Allen Salowe

Staying on Top of the Case

With all the new postoperative incidents confronting us, I thought it useful to start keeping a urologic diary. At first, these were just cryptic notes so that communications with the other team members would be more directly focused on recent experience and to help maximize their efficiency. Later, I prepared a one-page bulleted summary each month to keep track of key turning points, to sharpen the doctor's and PA's understanding of changes in my condition of healing, and to help document patient records.

Maintaining a journal can be an important activity for both the patient and the physician. First, the doctor has only limited time to grasp a few details when the patient comes to the clinic. The more persons that information must pass through, the greater the chance for error or misinterpretation. Second, the more directed and factual the information provided to the doctor and staff, the more efficiently and effectively they are able to employ their precious time.

Looking back, I marvel at the Mayo Clinic staff: the secretaries, nurses, PAs, and doctors. The Mayo Clinic is a large multispecialty group practice, but they are the best I have seen in *any* organization in taking a telephone message, *accurately* passing along that message, and the appropriate person acting on it. The size of the organization is not the issue; having good systems in place, operated by well-trained persons who *care for* the patient as a person is the difference. They need no endorsement from me, but clearly, Dr. William J. Mayo's counsel to doctors and staff, "The best interest of the patient is the only interest to be considered," takes on greater meaning in today's economics-driven health care environment.

Health provider organizations need to strive for a high degree of patient-focused quality. The discipline of medical coaching and collaborative medicine—patient-focused health care based on the principle of *fitness for use as judged by the user, the patient*—is introduced in Chapter 8. It is the new standard of quality that reaches beyond the classic industry definitions.

Health provider organizations are deliberately brought together to accomplish some *explicit* purpose. Health provider facilities exist to accomplish specific objectives. When achieved, those objectives represent the "value added," as economists call it, for the cost of operating the clinics, doctors' offices, and hospitals.

The act of caring in a formal health care organization cannot be

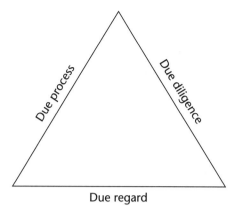

Figure 6   Holistic patient care, or due care, requires three elements: due regard, due process, and due diligence.

left to chance. Unfortunately, in health provider organizations at present, it is too often left to chance. Disciplined caring is accomplished through the exercise of *due care,* holistic patient care. As advanced by Leon Lessinger, the exercise of due care requires *due process, due diligence, and due regard,* which may be envisioned as an equilateral (equal-sided) triangle (Figure 6).

- *Due regard* serves as the base of the triangle. It symbolizes the motivational nature of patient care: to consider the patient in a way that reflects concern and affection. It is possible to master due regard by practicing its parts: accurate empathy, nonpossessive warmth, and authentic interest. Thus due regard is the foundation of the discipline of caring—to treat the patient as a person.
- *Due process* is one of the equal sides of the triangle. In the context of patient-centered care it means applying the principles of good practice—knowledge of expectations, knowledge of assistance, knowledge of results, knowledge of correction, and knowledge of a new start. These are also the fundamentals of the business principles of management by objectives (MBO).
- *Due diligence* is the other equal side of the triangle. Health care demands constant vigilance, to follow the steps that an ordinary and prudent person would take to help the patient heal. It calls for persistent effort, diagnosis and prescription, and corrective action.

Through the systemic exercise of due care, health care providers can establish the practice that links them with the care of the patient in the truest sense: to help the patient heal, to grow, and to fulfill. The synergy of meaning creates an unassuming but heart-felt result—caring for the patient and family.

Mental Transitions

While recovering from my third procedure in 6 weeks, I kept close track of my voiding—the time of the event and the measured amount. Perhaps it was just my way of celebrating that I was back on my own and that the TURP procedure had gotten things going naturally again. Maybe it was a way that the nurses found to keep me busy and out of trouble.

Norman Cousins stated, "The highest exercise of a physician's skills is to prescribe not just out of the little black bag but out of his or her knowledge of the human healing system. The ability of the physician in unblocking or enhancing or augmenting this healing system will constitute the grand confluence of the art and science of medicine."

A mysterious but important function is the way the body attends to its own healing. The body manufactures hair (for most of us), notwithstanding the onslaught of television commercials about hair restoration, maintains flexible and stretchable skin, grows new gum tissue, heals a bitten tongue, repairs fingernails, and on and on.

The urethra is composed of a most forgiving tissue and heals itself almost immediately after surgery, as does the bladder, which closes and heals its incision as soon as the postoperative suprapubic tube is removed. It is remarkable property of the body's healing system, which asserts its balances under adverse circumstances. It was time for me to allow the natural processes of healing to augment the efforts of the health provider team.

♦ **Taking Charge Advisory 18:** Let nature do some of the work.

Starting Over

It finally looked as though I was on my way to recovery and a measure of normalcy. My plumbing seemed to be functioning normally. As I left the hospital, my spirits were high. Leakage was minimal. When I got home I even felt well enough to try out my potency, and that worked pretty well, too.

I soon ventured out again from what had become a health care cocoon. I set up some lunches with business and personal friends and started back down the path toward normal living. One weekend Cynthia and I dared to go to the hardware store for some badly neglected home improvement supplies. Of all people, we ran into Mike Wehle, along with another Mayo Clinic urologist, browsing the plumbing department. It seems as though our paths were destined to cross.

At first everything felt strange. It was as though I had been on a trip to the moon and I had returned safely. Astronaut Frank Borman, Commander of the Apollo 8 moonlanding mission, is a member of the prostate cancer survivors club as well.

My view of the world had also changed pretty dramatically after these experiences. Things that seemed critical just 6 months earlier now seemed pretty trivial. Not long after, one of my clients called and talked with me about a business problem. It immediately struck me how much my perception of important matters had changed. After running a project *for my life* the past 9 months, the business crises confronting me that day seemed trivial by comparison. This is not to suggest that my client's business situations were not important; on the contrary, they talked of real-world issues. It was simply that what seemed an earth-shattering concern to the client now looked pretty manageable to me.

Within a few weeks, the blockages began to occur again. This resulted in the need for a series of monthly trips back to the clinic for cystoscopic and dilation procedures in which the doctor used an instrument to examine the bladder and to dilate (stretch) the urethra. The prostate was almost gone, healthy tissue was growing back in its place, and the bladder looked clear. But the remaining dead fibrous tissue continued to create havoc by plugging up the urethra with the material as it sloughed off.

One of the nurses (and by now I knew them all personally) put me through a self-catheterization demonstration. So for the next 6 months I intermittently used this tool to keep the urethral channel clear and to withdraw any clots or dead tissue. I think I got pretty proficient at handling it.

After a year, the healing area became scarred, which caused the channel to begin to close down the diameter of its opening. At one point I was unable to insert the catheter at all. There was no choice but to return to the operating room for three minor incisions to the prostate scar to restore normal urethral function. Until the scarring settled down, it was necessary for the doctor to cystodilate (use the cystoscope to enter and stretch) the scarred area to allow healing to take place to a preferred-size opening.

During one cystodilation procedure, following an incision into the remaining scar tissue, I became unusually tense and edgy. Frankly, the surgery had me feeling my best in more than a year. I hated to break the spell. I was already an old hand at this cystoscopic stuff by now and in fact had canceled a dental appointment to be at the Mayo Clinic for that day's adventure (an indication of where a dentist visit fits on my tolerance for pain scale). For some reason, though, I seemed to make things more difficult than usual by being unable to fully relax. At a critical point Dottie, a urologic nurse, took my hand and squeezed it, which immediately calmed my tension.

Therapeutic presence is the conscious intention to be present for another in a healing or helpful way. This process highlights the importance of encouraging and helping care providers to enhance their own health and potential. Truly, you cannot give what you do not have. This deliberate act of *caring for* the patient is one of the cornerstones of medical coaching and collaborative medicine.

♦ **Taking Charge Advisory 19:** Occupy the mind in turbulent times.

Accidents Will Happen

Everything was working again and I was once more on the mend. Attending an American Cancer Society support group meeting allowed me to help others find their way as I gained from other's experiences. Writing gave purpose to each day. Many new subjects were explored. Internet research kept me in touch with an exploding world of information. Reading opened new pathways of thinking. Contact with friends allowed the window on the world to stay open. Generally, there were opportunities to stay busy. But somehow, I was developing a disquieting feeling. Almost 18 months had now passed since I had started down this path.

Finally, one day while talking by phone with Bernice, Dr. Wehle's secretary, I was engulfed by a general feeling of depression. I completely lost it and started to cry. Over the past year or so I had had many spontaneous crying episodes. It is said that for each hour under anesthesia, crying may periodically occur for a month. I had accumulated 12 "frequent anesthesia hours," and the major reward was ridding my body of prostate cancer. It was inevitable that sooner or later some degree of depression would set in. The fact that I had continued to exert a significant degree of oversight and control over my case probably helped ward off an earlier bout with depression.

In relating a similar experience of a patient following a serious diagnosis, Norman Cousins noted, "What was most important was that he felt he was not consigned to a passive role but was able to work in tandem with his physician."

Within 2 hours, Mike Wehle called. He reassured me that this bout of depression was not all that unusual. After all I had been through, I was seeing a light at the end of the tunnel. He arranged for a Mayo Clinic psychiatrist to see me the next day.

What set off this feeling of depression? First, I had felt as though I was almost healed. Then, the inconvenience and awkwardness of incontinence recurred. My every hour now revolved around what my bladder wanted. Furthermore, it was increasingly frustrating to figure out where I would go from here with my work and my life.

I wrote a half-page summary of my background and the situation leading to this emotional event, as it now seemed to me, and gave it to the psychiatrist at the beginning of our meeting. In keeping with the mission of project managing my own case and the principles of medical coaching, the written abstract helped to set the stage for an incisive review with the doctor.

When I was a child, there never seemed to be time to stop for essential bodily functions, unless I was absolutely forced to do so. Children are always too busy doing more important things. And as an active traveling guy most of my business career, stopping to relieve myself had never been high on my agenda. "Keep going until you burst" is the man's motto. Now, after years of neglecting my bladder, two well-worn pieces of advice took on a new meaning: "Go with the flow" and "Look out for number one." I had to accept a new reality of partial incontinence and learn to adapt to and live with it. A colleague insists that the following quotations are attributable to Queen Victoria: "Never stand when you can sit," "Never walk when you can ride," and "Never pass up an opportunity to go to the bathroom."

♦ **Taking Charge Advisory 20:** Listen to your body.

After all of this, it appeared that things were going my way. More than a year and a half into this saga, my PSA remained undetectable (lower than 0.1). The prostate was finally gone, truly obliterated from the body by cryosurgery. My plumbing system was working fairly normally again, and I no longer needed to poke myself with a thin tube. I felt fairly good, although I still tired too easily, in my opinion.

On the other hand, incontinence continued. And, on occasion, there was an embarrassing moment, one of those accidents that only mother nature could spring. This caused great personal consternation. It was all but impossible to return to my business. But among friends, these occasional mishaps became easier to live with. It was necessary to perform under new ground rules, dictates legislated by and governed by the body. Surprisingly, acceptance generated new feelings of confidence and control.

♦ **Taking Charge Advisory 21:** Adapt to a new lifestyle.

Keeping Ahead of the Problem Curve

One of the toughest parts of project managing your own medical case is not being able to anticipate from one day to the next how you will feel. In truth, no one really can. It is just that until a medical condition emerges, we routinely take our good health and good fortune for granted.

Periodically keeping in touch with the Mayo Clinic urologic nurse, Diane, proved invaluable. She acted as a clearinghouse for questions or concerns to be shared with Dr. Wehle. The nurse knew a great deal about my case, and this increased the quality time with the doctor. Had it diminished the doctor's effectiveness? Thus far, not that I can tell.

At first, I seemed to continually pester Dr. Wehle's secretary, Bernice, with questions and she was a good sport about it. When my inquiries became more specific, Bernice would have Diane call me to explore my symptoms in greater depth before passing on her observations to the doctor. Sometimes it turned out to be more of a technical problem that could be handled by a PA. For the exchange of information to be effective, the health care provider must ask the right questions and the patient must be prepared to provide useful information to help focus the physician's response. My professional team was top-notch.

At present, the mission is to monitor what my body is trying to tell me. It is as though there are a series of "smoke detectors" in the body that periodically tell the brain how it is going. The patient's job is to integrate these signals with other factors and translate these signals for improved self-care or in further treatment by the health care team.

Extending the Time Spans

As healing has progressed, the intervals between postoperative treatments have also lengthened. PSA monitoring has remained scheduled on a 3-month basis.

Follow-up is essential. A person is never really out of the woods with this sort of thing. PSA levels have been known to rise after several years of remaining in the normal range. Cancer may mount an attack in another area of the body. Vigilance is imperative.

Keeping a Sense of Humor

One of the healthiest attributes a person can have is the ability to laugh fully and heartily at one's dilemmas. Surprise is a major ingredient of humor; Hollywood built an entire industry on this principle.

Laughter is the mind's way of dealing with something unexpected and incongruous.

A sense of humor has made a great deal of difference in my ability to deal with challenging and often stressful situations. It has helped me heal. The power of humor, in part, comes from involving yourself in a situation that can be perceived as amusing. Humor breaks the tension and reduces nervousness.

After my earlier infection and protracted hospital stay, I lost 20 pounds in a month. During the next visit to the clinic I quipped, "OK, I've completed the Jenny Craig crash program. Now what?" I highly recommend the healing power of laughter and the ability to see your situation through the prism of humor.

Today, I have one of those trendy sport-utility vehicles. This kind of transportation is really out of character for me. I neither hunt nor fish; I do not tow a boat and I have no need to go off-road four-wheeling. Our only need for a truck is Cynthia's penchant for bringing home another tree or trays of flowers to plant in her garden. She knows that "to plant a garden is to believe in tomorrow." Although I am half wounded from prostate surgery, she insists that I should drive the "macho" truck.

The experience of prostate cancer brought Cynthia and me closer together than ever. And our children (her two and my three) were convinced before that we were already joined at the hip. After all, we spent an inordinate amount of time together. Although I could sense the strain she was under, we laughed and enjoyed our new-found sense of love. We have rediscovered the fact that every moment is indeed precious. Perhaps no other experience could have had quite the same effect on us.

Keeping Good Records

No health care project can be complete without looking at the bookkeeping side of the story. It is no surprise that treating and healing prostate cancer is a serious financial commitment. Considering the alternatives, it is very cost effective. Sharing a few business housekeeping practices may prove helpful in tracking your own program.

First, it is highly advisable to keep a ledger of dates of service, charges, and insurance reimbursements, if applicable. By keeping my own set of records it made it much less stressful to reconcile differences with the hospital, the clinic, and the insurance carrier when necessary. With the amount of activity (six hospital stays, two trips to the emergency department, 40-plus clinic visits, seven outpatient procedures, and dozens of tests), plenty of opportunities arose for error—and each entity came in for its share of mistakes. Differences were much easier to resolve with good record keeping. Project management includes watching the business aspects as well.

Next, our insurance carrier, as do most, use the "ordinary and customary" standard, as determined by treatment code and zip code, to derive reimbursement amounts. The clinic frequently categorizes *multiple procedures* under a single code. On several occasions the clinic provided a copy of the doctor's operating report to the insurance carrier to help reconcile the differences. Similarly, hospital emergency department charges were challenged and clarified. On one occasion the clinic inadvertently charged for a cystoscopic procedure on two successive days and the carrier paid for it. I knew that there was no way I could possibly forget two of those things in a row. The documentation was subsequently corrected. Considering the numbers of patients involved, the enormous number of line items dealt with, and the complex coding systems used, it is remarkable that there are so few clerical errors.

An Unfinished Story

At this writing it has been more than 3 years since my prostate cancer experience began. There is good news as well as still-unfinished business. First, the good news. My PSA level remains at <0.1 (undetectable). I remain on 6-month recall to monitor that number, and I hold my breath each time the laboratory report results are brought up on the computer.

There is some unfinished business. Incontinence was a definite postoperative side effect. Scar tissue formed at the point where the internal sphincter muscle and prostate gland had previously been joined to one another. It was as though a sink washer had been damaged and needed replacement. The external sphincter, by contrast, was weak but still in good working order. With the help of computer-monitored electrostimulus biofeedback, the bladder calmed down and with the help of Kegel exercises the external sphincter regained its normal strength and effectiveness for holding urine.

I had two surgical options to try to repair my "sink washer" problem: an artificial sphincter implant or collagen injections. The artificial sphincter is placed surgically; its cuff surrounds the bladder neck and urethra and squeezes shut, compressing and blocking any urine leakage. The device is activated and deactivated by a pump placed in the scrotum. Collagen is a protein extract of connective tissue from cattle and is commonly used by plastic surgeons in a "face lift" to add shape or fullness. Three or four weeks before receiving this injection, the patient is given a skin test to assess any allergic reaction.

I opted for a collagen injection. I was placed under general anesthesia, and the collagen was injected through a flexible needle into the tissues at the bladder neck. When the procedure is successful, it causes the tissues to enlarge and squeeze together to prevent leakage. It is not uncommon for multiple injections to be needed to stabilize the treatment with the proper amount of material, and this method should retain its effectiveness for at least a few years. After two collagen injections there was noticeable improvement if I was not too active. Although at times discouraged, I persisted and, after the fourth collagen treatment, I was completely dry. Triumph!

Impotence is another story. Thus far erectile function, the ability to achieve an erection, is not as adequate as I might prefer. All aspects of prostate cancer treatments can have an effect on erections. Radical prostatectomy, cryosurgery, and radiation can each damage the complex of nerves and blood vessels that allow a man to achieve and maintain an erection.

The ability to function sexually in part helps define a man's role in the world as he sees it. It is no wonder, then, that the loss of erectile ability can have a deep effect on a man. Many men with erectile dysfunction suffer emotionally, often silently. They may tell themselves, "If I can't have normal sex with my partner, I'm a failure as a man and a lover." Or they may worry, "Will she leave me if I can't satisfy her needs?" Such feelings may result in anxiety, despair, self-consciousness, anger, guilt, and lack of fulfillment.

Both partners are affected by the emotions associated with erectile dysfunction. It is not uncommon for men to make excuses or sidestep sexual situations with their partners in an effort to avoid confronting this dysfunction. These actions can make a woman feel inadequate in the relationship, making *her* often feel rejected, lonely, and depressed.

Thus a man's failure to talk about his condition may contribute to a woman's feelings of anxiety or depression.

How has all of this affected Cynthia and me? We have enjoyed a very close and loving relationship in our 20 years of marriage. We started with a torrid love affair and built our structure of commitment and caring along the way. Faced with the realities of prostate cancer, we knew the consequences (life or death) and set our priorities at the outset. Life together, for as long as we could make it, was number one to us both. Quite honestly, at times I have become a bit dejected as I contemplated what has happened to our rich sex life. But Cynthia has repeatedly calmed me, and together we are building a new and richer answer to this aspect of our lives. As incontinence was brought under control, we turned our attention to the many ways now available for dealing with impotence, including devices, injection, and medications.

Remember my friend Lou? He's OK now. But one of his older farmer friends, age 72, decided to try the injection method to stimulate erection. He also concluded that if a small amount of injection material was good, a lot would be even better. Three hours after a self-injection, he walked, a bit bent over, into the local hospital and asked if they could make his erection go down.

Connecting With Other Survivors

I read once that there exists a fellowship among those who bear the mark of pain. I experience this whenever I attend a Man to Man meeting or when I get a call from a man now considering his prostate cancer treatment alternatives in the face of uncertain results.

For those who are distant from this fraternity, there is great difficulty in understanding what lies beneath the pain. I have listened to and seen first hand the fear, anguish, and doubt among my fellow survivors as well as those just beginning the long, dark journey into treatment and healing. Some talk frankly about matters among themselves that they admittedly would never pursue with their doctor. In my case:

- A feeling of peril and vulnerability that comes from having a serious disease
- The knowledge that one stray cancer cell can eventually kill me
- The underlying fear of never being normal again—physically and sexually

- A reluctance to be viewed as a complainer
- A wish not to worry my loved ones and family
- The battle—wanting to be left alone and yet the terror of being apart
- A conspicuous loss of self-esteem
- A feeling that illness, especially prostate cancer, resonates inadequacy
- The fear of decisions being made behind my back
- The need to know more, yet dreading the knowing
- Notwithstanding prior experience, the fear of invasive technologies
- The periodic test updates and the anxiety of what the data might say this time
- An underlying hostility toward those poking me for blood
- The torment of facing big, inhuman-scaled machines with flashing lights and a person talking to me through a microphone
- A constant desire for the warmth and reassurance of human contact: Cynthia sitting at the side of my bed holding my hand; a nurse's warm smile; the doctor or PA checking back on my progress
- A need to speak openly to other prostate cancer survivors about private matters

I know that I have been lucky. By the slender threads of fate, I wound up being in the right place at the right time with the finest team of health care providers one could possibly imagine. It all began when I decided that the experts needed the patient as a teammate. And as I have not-so-subtly hinted, I hope that they have looked on my active participation and project management as a new beginning.

Chapter 8

Medical Coaching and Collaboration

with Leon M. Lessinger, Ed.D.

I can still remember our family doctor coming to our house for a bedside examination when I was a child. In his small black bag he carried the barest of instruments: a thermometer, a stethoscope, a blood pressure cuff, bandages, and other simple devices. The doctor relied heavily on clues from my mother and from me, the patient. He took the time to ask many questions and listened carefully. He completed his examination, stated his diagnosis, and then phoned in a prescription to be delivered from the neighborhood druggist's. Our doctor always took the time to be warm and reassuring.

As we approach a new century, things have certainly changed. Health care providers now function in the "Information Era," that moment in history when "high tech" has become the expected norm, when what patients increasingly need is "high touch," the human side of medicine, which is so essential to healing. Time has joined disease as the enemy of the health care provider. In fact, disease always has time on its side. Physicians struggle against economic pressures while better armed than ever with new technologies and tools.

Together with Dr. Leon Lessinger, Eminent Scholar in Education Policy and Economic Development, we have worked for some time to define the concept and tools for implementing *medical coaching,* or perhaps more appropriately, *medical collaboration.* Dr. Lessinger is a licensed psychologist who previously served with others, including Norman Cousins, as a Clinical Professor of Medicine at UCLA.

To merely see technology primarily as only a way to either reduce costs or accelerate output is painfully simplistic: Technology is really a means for creating productive human environments.

New Opportunities for the Patient

Collaborative environments have to be created. When you shut a door, you do not get privacy, you shut out people. The critical difference between communication and communicative collaboration is that collaboration is supposed to produce something. Collaboration is a relationship. At its very heart is a desire or need to solve a problem or create or discover something within a set of constraints.

Information introduces new opportunities for patients to become their own healers and for health care providers to help facilitate new levels of patient self-awareness. Improving the quality of health care in an era of spiraling health care costs, managed care, and diagnostic-related group payment plans leaves only one economically viable alternative—to increase the effective involvement of the patient in each of the four stages of health care:

- Diagnosis, including improved self diagnosis
- Proactive patient-physician interaction
- Full participation in treatment selection
- Active responsibility for effective posttreatment

Information Is the Iron Link

Patients and health providers interface at a very narrow point. Similar to two space modules carefully linking up in space at high speed, patient and health care providers "dock" together precisely during a very brief time span. During this critical event, the health care providers must effectively withstand time pressures. Patients are concerned with quickly and clearly communicating primary and secondary symptoms.

In a compressed time period, the health care provider listens, learns, and leads the patient in a specific direction—sometimes prematurely. The opportunity to improve health care delivery and quality rests, in part, with coupling the self-help movement with the tools and perceptions of the information era.

The Critical Assumption

Prevention is still the cheapest and most effective way to treat any illness.

- No one can take better care of you than you.
- The patient must be an active player in his own self-care as well as in his or her own health care decisions.
- It is not the insurance carrier but the *patient* who is the consumer of health care services.

In prostate cancer, the next best thing to prevention is to detect the cancer early. Only the man, with his loved one's help, can accomplish this.

The Benefits of Improved Information

For health care providers, information management provides new opportunities to increase delivery effectiveness as well as to avoid and reduce the costs of nonessential services.

For patients, there are abundant opportunities to improve preventive health care. In turn, this can lead to lowering family costs, helping to maintain long-term earnings potential, which helps to accrue economic wealth, and to lower family insurance costs.

Central Issues in Health Care

The central issue in health care is to set the stage for and to help devise the conditions that support an individual's own healing process and that encourage the active interaction and participation of patients, families, and professional caregivers.

Health care is presently operating in a near-crisis mode. It is a time of shrinking reimbursements, intense competition, rapid technologic advances, and growing consumer uncertainty.

Reform plans among health insurance and health provider networks share a common theme: to foster technologic improvement in traditional health care and to induce managed competition to drive down health care costs. Policy makers, health care providers, and insurance payment plans are in an economic tug of war. This approach to sharpening today's economy-driven health care system may jeopardize its primary purpose: to create an interactive healing system in which both patients and health care professionals team up to heal the body, mind, and spirit of persons who are ill.

Gathering Information

Medical coaching helps the patient learn how to accumulate the right information, that is, facts that will facilitate better decision making. There is no shortage of advice and counsel. On-line services, the Internet, and the World Wide Web are already inundating us with vast amounts of electronic data, but not all of it is useful or reliable. The *Healthwise Handbooks* (Healthwise, Inc., Boise, Idaho) and the *Mayo Clinic Family Health Book* (in both a single-volume, 5-pound version and on CD-ROM) are good home sources of information. Patient empowerment is available through information technology, but only if health care providers play a role in guiding the patient in the proper directions.

The Patient's View

To the patient, medicine is historically a curative process: antibiotics to treat bacterial infections, corrective topical treatments for skin conditions, and so on. Medication only helps knock out the infection and surgery removes an unwanted growth. In all cases the object of health care is to help put the patient in the best condition for natural healing to occur. Information and a positive frame of mind played pivotal roles in the project management of this prostate cancer case.

The Self-Fulfilling Prophecy

It is important to understand how you may unwittingly create a self-defeating mental image. Our mental "scripts" and "videos" of how a health crisis will be resolved can actually produce physical conditions and lead to actions that are in accord with our thoughts and images. Energy follows thought. If I visualize myself as being in good health, chances are more favorable that I will truly be in good health. If I imagine that I am going to get (or be unable to shake off) some dreadful disease, I increase the odds that this will happen. If you believe something will happen, you both consciously and unconsciously act in ways that create the prophesied event.

The consequences of negative thinking are reflected in what Janette Rainwater calls the "jack story":

Once upon a time a man driving on a little-traveled road in the desert suddenly had a flat tire. To his consternation, he realized that he had no jack to raise his car and change the tire. Then he remembered that he had passed a service station about 5 miles back, and started walking. And thinking. "You know, way out here in the desert there are no other stations around. If the man who owns it doesn't want to be helpful, there's no other place I can go. I'm really at this guy's mercy. He could skin me good just for lending me a jack so I can change my tire. He could charge me $10 . . . $20 . . . why that SOB! My God, how some people will take advantage of their fellow man!" The man arrives at the service station. The owner comes out and asks in a friendly way, "Hello, what can I do for you?" And our friend shouts, "You can take your goddamned jack and shove it!"

There are two solutions to avoid falling into the trap of a jack story. First, what is happening right now? What am I doing? What am I feeling? What am I thinking? Second, what do I want for myself in this new moment? Do I want to continue? Do I want to make some changes? In becoming mindful of your situation, you have made a decision to change.

Concentrating on Patient Self-Help

It is now time to concentrate on a dimension of health care heretofore recognized for its curative value but undervalued for its economic benefits: to prepare, instruct, counsel, involve, and guide the patient through the diagnostic and posttreatment stages of healing. In an age of high-tech, high-touch health care, the economic and human benefits of improving patient-directed pretreatment and posttreatment are several:

- The ability to continuously monitor changes in health—listening to your body and responding appropriately
- Developing the sensitivity to identify direct and indirect symptoms at the earliest stages and to sharpen your ability to communicate observations more clearly to your doctor
- Creating a preventive maintenance *mind-set* toward your own health

Improved self-directed health care has become essential—both economically critical and physiologically indispensable. The traditional health care system is overloaded; it remains largely focused on improving efficient delivery of patient services. Patients can be empowered to grasp methods and benefits of self-directed health care, to apply proven routines of self-monitoring and early self-diagnosis, and to more clearly communicate to doctors and other health care providers the symptoms of their health difficulties.

The Meaning of Change

The basic tool of healing is self-observation. It is important to master the difference between accurate self-observation and abnormal or obsessive introspection, a form of squirrel-cage thinking.

Change occurs when you become what you are, not when you try to become what you are not. Change does not occur by resolves to do better, by trying harder, or by demands from others.

Change seems to happen when you abandon the chase after what you want to be (or think you should be) and accept—and fully experience—what you are.

Improving self-care. Television advertising has assumed a greater role in educating patients to the symptoms of common conditions and the potential cures to be had through over-the-counter medications. Awareness campaigns are routinely trying to better inform patients of their potential risk of life-threatening disease.

Programs to increase public knowledge concerning prostate cancer and breast cancer are but two leading campaigns aimed at men and women. Regrettably, sound-byte medicine is no more valuable or effective in building understanding than is sound-byte politics. The tip of the iceberg is *not* what sank the Titanic.

Patient options. The physician can only prescribe a course of treatment based on his or her cumulative and present knowledge. The physician has a tough enough job just keeping pace with developments and changes in the practice of medicine. It is scarcely a stretch to estimate that the weekly amount of new information available to a physician today far exceeds what was read in a year of medical school. The principal *software* of medical coaching, when routinely used, may be expected to advance the everyday practice of medicine.

Building patient independence. Health care providers are keenly aware of the need to *wean* patients and get them functioning on their own. Medical coaching serves three main purposes. First, it better equips the patient and doctor to jointly address the matter at hand efficiently and effectively. Second, self-generated information helps to further *sensitize* the patient to specific incidents of self-monitoring and more effective self-care. Third, better information helps document the patient record so that both the patient and physician are supplied current ongoing data.

Patient self-healing. Medical coaching encourages the patient to take an active role in self-healing, both directly and indirectly. The process of information gathering promotes participatory thinking and spawns information that can be acted on. Further, a shift in focus and perspective takes place in the patient's mind as he or she becomes *more directly* involved in discerning and monitoring his or her own condition. This activity discourages that scourge of wellness, hypochondria.

Health care and aging. To overcome generalizations about aging, it is virtually impossible to escape a great deal of propaganda about our supposed loss of power as we get older. People see themselves as deteriorating as they get older. We have been told that this is an incontrovertible fact of life; that the human body was not made to function for the length of time the average person lives today. In reality, however, unless a person suffers from a disease such as Alzheimer's, most older people do not need to lose their mental powers. As for physical powers, the body can be kept lithe, strong, and sexual into old age. What is required, though, is practice. "Use it or lose it" is still good advice.

Improved patient healing. With self-training through medical coaching, a person can soon observe genuine mastery of the healing process. People with such mastery exude an observable energy and poise. Interaction with someone like that makes us feel better, and we are then better able to foster our own healing experience.

Patient advocates. Recently, hospitals have increasingly appointed patient advocates out of concern that the patient's best interest be represented at such times as the patient is unable to properly perform this function himself. Medical coaching helps transform a quasilegal advocate's role into a positive healing one.

Centering the Experiences of Health Care Providers

It is through the experiences of the patient that the health care provider gains the greatest insight into diagnosis and the effectiveness of previously administered treatments. Medical coaching helps center these experiences in the form of usable information that can be acted on.

The patient-physician linkage. Forging a strong patient-physician bond yields tangible benefits to both. The patient feels in control of his or her own destiny; the doctor gains the cooperative participation of the patient—the most important working member of the team. This union synergizes to benefit the patient's health and the efficiency and effectiveness of the physician.

Preventive health care. It remains no secret that the shortest distance to good health is through preventive (wellness) health care. Why is it so difficult for an idea that is so seemingly logical and effective to take hold? First, dollars that move through the health care system do so in payment for diagnosis and treatment. Few provisions are made for payment to health care providers for rendering advice and prevention. Second, nowhere is time more precious than in health care. Minutes spent educating the patient on improved self-monitoring can help pay great future dividends. Regrettably, the health care system rewards fire fighting, not fire prevention.

One exception is the annual physical examination, which is today being partially reimbursed by more insurance carriers. It is through just such an opportunity that a combination prostate screening test turned up my case of locally advanced stage prostate cancer. My wife's routine self-examinations and annual mammography evaluations helped to provide screening for detection of her early-stage breast cancer.

Improving patient knowledge. There is no shortage of reading and video material available on health topics. Since I began to write this story, the amount of health care information available on the Internet has expanded geometrically. Chapter 9, Patient Empowerment Through Information, provides some examples of presently available Internet information related to prostate cancer—some of it good, some not so good.

The value of information is determined in part by its content as well as its timeliness. A better approach to patient education and training is through integrating it into the *routine* operations of the physician's or clinic's daily work. The need becomes increasingly apparent as larger and more elaborate managed care facilities and organizations become the standard in U.S. health care.

Increasing treatment effectiveness. Physicians already recognize that treatment is more than medical science. It includes the full participation of the patient in a mind-body relationship. Much is known about this phenomenon and how it works. But the threshold event is to draw the patient into a *participatory* role in the healing process. Medical coaching proposes marrying information technologies with routine segments of today's system of provider services.

Patient-physician collaboration. Not all physicians welcome the full involvement of the patient. This will change as patients demand greater accountability for their health care dollars. In place of a defensive view of patient inclusion, the full patient-physician partnership can blossom into a new win-win result for both. A direct product of medical coaching and collaboration can also be more effective documentation.

Facilitating patient awareness. Educators have known for years that the best way to learn is to teach. Involving the patient in self-monitoring helps move the patient measurably farther up the scale of self-awareness. Medical coaching encourages the patient to seize the opportunity to remain actively involved in his or her own health care.

Educating the doctor. It is up to the patient to keep the doctor informed. Even subtle changes that ordinarily would not merit a thought should be routinely monitored by the patient, then effectively communicated to the doctor. Most men know the warning signals for a severe heart attack—pain down the left arm, the feeling of a steel plate pressing on the chest. But when those late symptoms arise, the patient may be only minutes from death. The warning signals of prostate disease are equally subtle and often ignored—increased urinary urgency and frequency and mild discomfort. Well in advance of a major quake, the body, like the earth, sends out many small seismic signals that need to be learned and heeded.

The medical diary. It takes little effort to jot down key events or changes in your health. It may prove essential in helping the physician come to a more accurate diagnosis and appropriate course of treatment. Medical coaching diaries have proved successful in such wide-ranging situations as helping diagnose a rare case of Kawasaki disease in a 1-year-old child, quickly updating a psychiatrist with possible sources of depression, postoperative pain from neck surgery, rescheduling urethral dilation in postoperative prostate treatment, and weight control programs.

Results From New Efforts

It might be said that a person is a person because of other people. If you grow up with this perspective, your identity is based on the fact that you are seen—that the people around you respect and acknowledge you as a person.

Current medical practice, technologically filtered and under inordinate time pressures, too often violates this. Patients are known to complain that "the doctor doesn't see me as a person; I'm simply a body part—an object for intervention, not a whole, feeling, and spiritual person." Too often, medical practice is body part medicine.

The great physicians of the past understood that the secret in the care of a person is to *care for* that person. Caring for a person is a form of stewardship. If I care for you, I see myself as serving your interests, your welfare, your wellness. The magic of healing stems from the phrase *cared for.* The secret in the care of a patient is to *care for* the patient.

Building Mutual Trust

A healer is a person who intentionally helps someone grow both intellectually and emotionally. This help is made possible and encouraged by the creation of a caring, humane, trusting, and compassionate environment. We can start with a simple fact. We need only a person willing to listen. If that person learns to accept and encourage additional dialogue, we have made a striking advance in applying the tools of medical collaboration.

Walter Menninger, founder of the Menninger Foundation, once stated, "There are numerous examples of physicians who are absolutely superb technicians, with all the latest knowledge and skill, but who approach patients in such a cold manner as to prompt doubt and distress. Members of medical society boards of censors are keenly aware that patients are often so unhappy with that kind of care that they file a formal grievance. In the investigation of such complaints, it becomes clear that, more often than not, the breakdown has been in the 'caring' aspect of the physician-patient relationship—not in the quality of technical care and treatment provided."

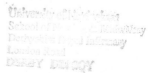

Chapter 9

Patient Empowerment Through Information

Finding Useful Answers

Knowledge is power for the patient, and information is its source of energy. The traditional sources of information identified by A.F.U.D./Gallup as most often used by prostate cancer patients were listed in Chapter 6. In subsequent chapters some of the ways that you and your family might use the new electronic information technologies to supplement more traditional prostate cancer information sources were identified.

Much of what I learned came through collaboration with my colleague, Frank Schnidman, presently Visiting Professor of Law at the University of Miami. We also serve together as Senior Fellows of the Florida Center for Electronic Communications of the Florida State University System, located at Florida Atlantic University. Frank is also cofounder of the American Center for Patient Decision Making (ACPD), a not-for-profit resource for medical information supporting a patient's health care decisions, located on the Internet at *www.decision.org*.

It takes digging and persistence to find *useful* answers to tough health care questions. Some of what I turned up proved beneficial in furthering my own health education; it better equipped me for coming to grips with some tough decisions. On the other hand, some of the sources and quality of information ranged from disappointing to distressing.

Here are some general findings to help you on your journey. Remember, use these information sources to *supplement* your local library, bookshop, your doctor who you know and trust, and the more traditional sources listed in Chapter 6.

Don't be misled by data moving through cyberspace. All roads lead back to your *physician-partner.*

What Is the Internet?

The Internet is a giant network of computers located all over the world that communicate with each other. A computer user with a modem (a computer device that allows direct connection to a telephone jack) can send a message electronically to another user across the country or around the world, and it will get there in seconds.

Once you have the equipment (minimally, a 14.4, or preferably, 28.8 BPS–speed modem and at least a 386-speed computer), you need to contact an Internet service provider, listed in the yellow pages as "Internet services" or "on-line services," to provide you a "ramp," so to speak, onto the information highway. These service providers generally charge a flat access fee per month, such as $19.95, for unlimited access time.

There are almost unlimited services for prostate cancer patients and survivors on the Net. There is electronic mail (e-mail). You can dial people, leave electronic messages on "electronic" bulletin boards, and meet new people with common interests. There are already a number of electronic prostate cancer support groups that can be reached on the major on-line services, such as America Online, CompuServe, Prodigy, and Microsoft Network, or directly by way of *browsing* (also called surfing or scanning) the Internet. Soon more will be available.

Originally, the Internet was set up by government and research institutions so that they could communicate with each other. Today individuals may access the Internet through the commercial on-line services mentioned or a local provider, as described. It is as easy as or maybe even easier than calling your local or long-distance carrier for telephone service.

Early on, one of my most productive search experiences came from logging onto the Library of Congress's site. There is no charge to use this vast source of research material. Today you can reach the Library of Congress on the Net at *http://lcweb.loc.gov/.*

In my early search for reliable confirmation of other information sources, I followed the on-screen instructions and took "the health path" to the National Institutes of Health and the National Cancer Institute. I was given a series of options and the related 800 (toll-free) phone numbers to request further written information. In only 3 days my mail box bulged with reliable information that immediately proved useful for cross-checking earlier findings and opening up new investigational paths that seemed promising. That was the way it was just 3 years ago.

Today I log on to my local provider, with whom I have a monthly service agreement, and I click on my Netscape Navigator or Microsoft Internet Explorer software to browse the Web, looking for the subject "prostate cancer." First, as soon as I am connected to the introductory home page, I type in *http://www.search.com* in the address box at the top. This takes me to a site provided by C/NET. This site provides me *no-charge access* to 25 powerful search engines. Search engines are tools that can be used to quickly scan every available Web page in the entire global library of electronic information. According to Digital Equipment Corporation, there are 15 billion words, 30 million pages on the Web so far. Using one of the three most powerful search engines, Alta Vista, Yahoo, and Magellan, I type in "prostate cancer" and click on search. Here's what happens:

1. Alta Vista lists the top 100 of 20,000 matching documents. The word *prostate* comes up more than 65,000 times, *cancer* 840,000 times. I review each for a match with my present interests, then click on those articles I want to peruse further.

2. Yahoo turns up more than 4000 documents that include the words *prostate cancer*. I review and click on the ones I want to read.

3. Magellan comes back with about 25,000 results rated by relevancy. The top 12 sites are presented. I click on each site for further information.

As you click on any one of the topics that look most promising to your search, it will in turn carry you to more and more information, some of it new, some duplications.

Keep in mind that you are not studying for a medical degree, nor are you planning to become board certified in urology. You are trying to collect information that you think will help you better understand your disease and act in your particular case.

The so-called "information superhighway" is becoming an increasingly important resource for all kinds of people. For the purpose of project managing a matter of serious health concern, it provides access to untold numbers of opportunities to learn and share the experiences of researchers, other patients, and their families. It may also accidentally lead you astray so be mindful, as you would in accumulating or using any other data. With these cautions in mind, here are some hints for expanding your electronic search for information that may prove relevant to your case or family's needs.

Remember, no one takes better care of you than you. Finding what you *want* as well as what you may *need* are distinctly different.

Using Multiple Information Sources

As stressed earlier, the information you find is *never* complete. Once you think you have an answer, *do not stop looking.* You may find more details, or a different answer to the same question. Do not stop because you find one source that seems to have the answer.

The Internet seems large (there are reportedly more than 20 million persons worldwide connected at this writing), but it is really composed of relatively tiny communities that do not always cross-pollinate. You are in charge of this project also.

The following is an alphabetic listing of the addresses of some prostate cancer Web sites I found particularly helpful; you too may find them useful. At least it is a start. All addresses are *case sensitive.* Watch those dots and the direction of slashes.

- Duke University Medical School: Prostate cancer updates.
  http://www.duke.edu/~ebc/prostate.html
- MedWeb: Biomedical Internet resources is maintained by Emory University.
  http://www.emory.edu/whscl/medweb.html
- Michigan Prostate Institute: One of the most thorough sites. Includes step-by-step explanation with diagrams of a radical prostatectomy. The Institute's Director was formerly Chief of Urology at Mayo Clinic.
  http://www.surg.med.umich.edu/urology/urology.m.prostate.i.html
- New York Times Syndicate: Provides links to recent prostate cancer articles. Go to Yad (Your Health Daily); Common topics: Cancer/Select prostate cancer.
  http://nytsyn.com/

- Northwestern Medical School: Access departments and go to a broad selection of information dealing with urology and prostate cancer.
  http://www.nums.nwu.edu/
- OncoLink: The University of Pennsylvania Cancer Resource. A very complete link to associated prostate cancer Web sites.
  http://www.oncolink.upenn.edu/disease/prostate/
- Prostate Cancer Home Page: A comprehensive source of information and services dedicated to prostate cancer patients and their relatives providing free, easy-to-understand information.
  http://prostate.com
- The Prostate Cancer Home Page of the University of Michigan Medical School: Bulletin board; protocol information; localized treatment options; research news; e-mail; physicians and scientists; links to other locations.
  http://www.cancer.med.umich.edu/prostcan/prostcan.html
- The Prostate Cancer Info Link: A fairly complete connection to prostate cancer information.
  http://www.comed.com/prostate/
- Prostate Pointers: Provides an extensive and detailed list of prostate cancer Web sites compiled by and maintained by a motivated and scientifically trained prostate cancer survivor.
  http://rattler.cameron.edu/prostate/prostate.html/
- The Prostatitis Foundation: An *Internet-only* resource for prostate cancer information; quite complete.
  http://www.prostate.org/
- Usenet: Access directly from *http://www.search.com.* Puts you directly in touch with information from prostate cancer patients and survivor discussion groups.
  alt.support.cancer.prostate
  sci.med.prostate.cancer

You Have to Give to Get

The best metaphor for the Internet culture is a cocktail party. People are willing to talk about themselves and their experiences, as long as the exchange is an interesting one. If it seems that you have done your homework and are trying to get answers to some final questions, you are likely to get a better reception than if it looks as though you are too lazy to go to the library.

Use the Whole Tool Kit

Serious inquiry calls for using the same line of research throughout all potential resources—news groups, mailing list archives, servers, and on-line databases. On-line services such as America Online, CompuServe, Prodigy, and Microsoft Network offer access to a great deal of information that has been organized and is not necessarily available on the Internet. If you omit any of these when looking for information, you are likely to get low-quality data.

I have found that men of the prime age group for prostate cancer (mostly over age 50 or even 60) are not generally users of electronic information sources. In fact, a recent C/NET survey showed that 80% of users on the Internet are between the ages of 18 and 44. Nonetheless, there are often inquiries from younger persons who are trying to help a father, an uncle, or a friend come to grips with the decision dilemmas presented by prostate cancer. You will as often give help as receive it. You will also benefit from giving these matters deeper thought, you will grow more secure in your use of the knowledge you have acquired, and you will be equipping yourself to make better informed decisions.

Build Your Own Road Map

It is essential to keep track as your search begins to lead you down different pathways. Like country lanes, information branches in all directions. Building our own database of useful notations and pointers is a constant and difficult effort, but an important one. You simply cannot depend on indices that other people have built to be good enough for your needs. *Bookmark* (placing an electronic bookmark is a tool on your browser) the most important sites that you visit so you can easily return to them.

The concept of each individual's prostate cancer being a statistical case of one is driven home when you talk with other patients directly, through books or through electronic media. But do not get discouraged; these distinctions only serve to highlight for you what may prove to be important differences in your specific case and thus will help point the way for your further attention.

Adapt as You Search

Although you begin by expressing your question a certain way, you must be ready and able to change directions to accommodate different viewpoints (remember the nine underlying principles of problem solving in Chapter 6 and Appendix B). For instance, you might first decide to look at news groups or lists for starters, yet later discover that a university is doing research in exactly the area of your interest. See what advice they offer.

Target Information Sources

There is nothing wrong with sending e-mail to someone asking for help, but you need to find the right person. That means doing some research. Recently, the 5-year-old son of some dear friends was diagnosed with Hallervorden-Spatz disease, a rare genetic disease affecting the brain. Through one of my directed searches I found my way to the National Organization for Rare Disorders, where I learned that only 70 cases are presently reported in the literature. A bit more data mining turned up the e-mail address of a doctor at the National Institutes of Health who has seen several patients and authored research papers on efforts to find the genetic link to prevention and cure. Within 48 hours he responded to my e-mail request for help.

If prostate cancer treatment is the subject you are interested in, find out who the important people are in the field and send them an e-mail. If you cannot find their e-mail addresses, call them on the phone and ask them. If anyone knows about the appropriate Internet resources you seek, it is someone in that field, not someone standing by when you electronically browse a news group.

The World Web has brought to the computer the *electronic catalog*. Some of the nation's leading medical institutions have generalized information available on this branch of the Internet. For example, some frequently asked questions have been adapted from the popular Mayo Clinic page, which can be reached on the Web at *http://www.mayo.edu*. This approach may prove useful to you in your own search and questioning.

- Why do patients come to this health provider organization? Do you need a referral?
- How soon are appointments available?
- Who presently owns this hospital? This health provider? Is it public, not-for-profit, or private, for profit?
- Does the hospital or organization specialize in certain areas?
- Does my doctor have admitting and surgical privileges?

- What important medical discoveries or innovations have originated here?
- How do costs compare with costs at other medical centers?
- If I am a member of a managed care plan, can I still get access to this hospital?
- How is health care reform affecting the hospital or health provider organization, and what is it doing to adapt to changes?

If you live near a major city, one or more major health care facilities or urologic specialty groups will likely be available to you. The technical editor of your local newspaper may be able to provide you with Web sites that also serve your area or region of the country. Once you reach the Web, a number of sources for quick-response general information can be accessed. For example, in the index, The Prostate Cancer InfoLink highlights the following:

- The location of your prostate and its functions
- The causes, symptoms, and prevention of prostate cancer
- Abbreviations for prostate-specific antigen (PSA), digital rectal examination (DRE), prostatic acid phosphatase (PAP), transrectal ultrasound (TRUS), and others
- Prostate cancer screening, early detection, and diagnosis of prostate cancer
- Clinical stages of prostate cancer and understanding Gleason scores
- Why there are no easy answers
- Treatment of prostate cancer: an overview, treatment of localized, locally advanced, and advanced prostate cancer
- Treatment of hormone-resistant prostate cancer
- Pharmaceuticals used to treat prostate cancer
- Prostate cancer frequently asked questions
- The prostate cancer experience; talking with your physician; what your family needs to know
- Prostate cancer support organizations
- Physicians experienced in the treatment of prostate cancer; where can you go to learn more?
- Prostate cancer dictionary

Once you enter the world of the Web, you will be introduced to many new sources of information. From time to time it may be advisable to refer to the nine underlying principles in Chapter 6 and Appendix B to help keep the cascading information in proper perspective.

Allow Enough Time

The night before you need an answer is not the time to start looking for data. If you are in a hurry, go to a library—not the Internet. Any in-depth search of the Internet takes time. It takes time for people to answer your questions, time for you to read through mailing list or news group archives, and time for things to filter their way around the world. Sometimes a week or two will pass before you hear back—the person who has your answer may only check in once a week, or your message may have been missed. Any serious research effort takes at least 2 weeks, and preferably a month.

Be Discerning

A support group can help provide emotional support. But remember, it is *not* a place to turn for competent medical advice. Recently, I read a posting on an America OnLine prostate cancer support group from a distraught prostate cancer patient who had a life decision to make the *next* day related to a very complex combination of diagnostic factors. The best advice I could offer was to get a second medical opinion to confirm his concerns with his present situation. A support group can help provide just that—emotional support. It is *not* a place to turn for qualified medical advice.

Be Critical

Like many other sources of data, the Internet is full of misinformation. Just because something is available by computer over the Internet *does not mean it is true.* News groups are notorious for being wildly incorrect and misleading. For example, in one evening I came across advice on the following cancer "remedies": violets, tofu, palmetto extract, red sauce on pasta, Chinese herbs for prostate cancer, a combination offer of crystals, and a clinical report on treating cancer from an unnamed source.

It is not that people typically intend to be wrong or mislead anyone; it is simply that they often are mistaken or premature in reaching certain conclusions. If you plan to gather facts on the Internet, especially facts related to your life and health, make sure they can be backed up with confirming research that can be accessed from other sources (especially non-Internet ones). This is especially true if the data are going to be used for something as important as beating prostate cancer. With these cautions in mind, Appendix D provides additional addresses that may provide some helpful information.

Be Gracious

When I think I am dealing with a friendly and pleasant person on the other end of the wire, I am more likely to take extra time to look for answers and to forward additional information as it comes in. When I send back an answer and get no reply, I am certainly not going to continue dumping matter into what looks like a black hole.

This holds especially true if you join a discussion group of other patients where you can post questions and seek friendly advice. The on-line server (the party who provides and maintains the linkage) allows you to talk with other survivors. It is used for information, education, and bonding with the prostate cancer community. More than just information, communication is empowering. To become a member of a prostate cancer discussion group:

1. Send an e-mail to *listserv@sjuvm.stjohns.edu.*
2. Leave the subject line *blank* or use single character if your e-mail program requires it.
3. Place the following *message* in the body of the mail: "subscribe Prostate First name Last name."
4. Wait for a return message providing confirmation instructions.
5. Follow confirmation instructions.

If Necessary, Throw in the Sponge

CAUTION: Not everything you needed to know is on the Internet.

One of the benefits of the Net is that you can cover a great deal of ground from your keyboard, but you cannot even come close to covering it all, and there are many duplications of information.

If you make a good, honest effort and cannot find what you need, do not be hardheaded and insist that it has to be there. Things show up and disappear in cyberspace for no rational reason, and you cannot do anything about it—so do not spend too much time looking for something that is not there.

Our experience, nevertheless, has been that the community of interests among those who share the battle against a life-threatening disease draws together very quickly. And the camaraderie and warm friendship flows from battling a common enemy—prostate cancer.

Finally, use information sources as a *supplement* to your care, *not* as a substitute. All roads lead back to your physician-partner.

Chapter 10

The Diet Connection

For me, concentrating on nutrition and stress management is like a reformed alcoholic preaching about temperance. For a good part of my life I have engaged in less than ideal eating habits. I'm a big fellow and I always thought I needed two hamburgers at the picnic, two hot dogs at the ball game, or that second portion at mealtime. At fast-food restaurants, a big hamburger with cheese, fries, and a shake was my automatic response to the question, "What'll you have?"

My prime years in the corporate world were filled with stress—big companies, important meetings, life or death decisions (so I thought, or was led to believe), and a boss or two with typical type A characteristics who fed on crisis management—all situations made to order to induce stress.

It was easy for me to fall into that same groove. I went to work early, came home late, took too many long business trips, and ate badly. My closet was filled with a wardrobe of clothes in different sizes, depending on where I was on the "scales" of stress and eating. I now realize that the growth in my girth and suit size was a metaphor for a change in my general health and, more specifically, the growth and mutation of prostate cancer within my body.

Ernst L. Wynder, M.D., founder and President of the American Health Foundation (AHF), suggested in a private letter that an alternative prostate cancer treatment could be nutritional. "This is a course that anyone over [the age of] 70 and those who are younger should be seriously considering as an adjunct to whatever treatment they undergo." Dr. Wynder's words set me to thinking further about the nutrition connection, a causal link with the incidence of the disease, as well as the potential for adjuvant therapy accompanying clinical prostate cancer treatment.

In addition, others have asked about preventive steps to thwart an individual prostate cancer event. Not surprisingly, my three sons were intensely interested in this question. In fact, any man with a direct family history of the disease should have a keen interest in prevention and screening. At the 1997 Annual Meeting of the American Urological Association (AUA) in New Orleans, physicians at the Cleveland Clinic reported that "prostate cancer tends to be more aggressive in men with a family history of the disease than men with no family history." Knowing that their situation is equally precarious, African-American men and their partners should seek preventive guidance, as available.

Is there reliable evidence that links nutrition to the prevention and potential adjuvant treatment of prostate cancer? Could such evidence, although still largely circumstantial but nonetheless growing, help patients, regardless of age, with prevention or, if needed, adjuvant treatment of prostate cancer?

In an October 1996 editorial published in the *Journal of Urology*, Dr. Wynder and William R. Fair, M.D., from the Memorial Sloan-Kettering Cancer Center, strongly suggest that "We should consider that if invasive prostate cancer would be as uncommon in the United States as it is in Japan, and China, the mortality of prostate cancer would be of relatively minor concern to the oncological community and public at large."

Growth Cycle of Prostate Cancer

The progression of prostate cancer has already been strongly linked to dietary factors. To reasonably consider when and how decisions about diet might benefit all younger men, as well as the older prostate cancer patient, it is helpful to briefly review the process of tumor development in stages (a more complete description with effective color diagrams appears in an article entitled "How Cancer Arises" by Robert A. Weisenberg in the *Scientific American*).

- All men as they age experience some enlargement of the prostate gland. At the benign (noncancerous) stage, the normal prostatic cells reproduce too much (hyperplasia). Benign prostatic hyperplasia (BPH) eventually results when the enlarged prostate squeezes the urethra, the tube that carries urine from the bladder out through the penis, inhibiting or even restricting a normally strong urine stream. Relief is obtained through drug therapy or one of several surgical treatments to relieve pressure on the urethral tube.

- The affected prostate cells may multiply excessively and some may take on an abnormal shape and orientation (the tissue is said to exhibit dysplasia). Once again, with time, a rare mutation that alters cell behavior may occur.
- The affected cells may then become still more abnormal in growth and appearance. If the tumor has not yet broken through any boundaries between tissues (in situ cancer), it may remain contained indefinitely. However, some cells may eventually acquire additional mutations. It is in situ cancer that is most universally found at autopsy in American men who have died of other causes in their eighties and nineties.
- The progression from in situ cancer to invasive cancer of the prostate comes as the tumor invades the underlying tissue and sheds cells into the blood or lymph system. The mass is considered to have become malignant. The cancer may still be confined to the prostate capsule but the renegade cells are determined to establish new tumors (metastases), first to the adjacent lymph nodes and then throughout the body. These become lethal by disrupting vital organs.

In other words, the incidence of this disease increases with age and there is widespread prevalence of this disease found at autopsy in older American men. Taken together it strongly suggests that the cumulative effect of dietary factors is to act as a *cancer promoter* during the natural history of prostate cancer growth, and any resultant subsequent mortality.

What We Know About Diet and Prostate Cancer

On a worldwide scale there appears to be a strong correlation between prostate cancer death rates and fat consumption. The incidence of clinical prostate cancer is low in Asian men and higher in Scandinavian men. It is not that Swedish men are obese, but rather that the binders used to hold together those tasty foods on a smorgasbord table are high in fat content. Incidence rates vary 120-fold between

Chinese men and African-American men living in San Francisco. Although it is unclear whether this incidence can be explained by genetic or environmental factors, numerous studies show that men tend to take on the cancer risk of their host countries. For example, second-generation Japanese-American men exhibit the same prostate cancer characteristics as all other American men.

African-American men have a higher incidence of the disease than black Africans, notwithstanding the high profile cases of South Africa's President Nelson Mandela and Zaire's (now Congo) former late president Mobutu. In the period 1978 to 1981 the prostate cancer incidence rate of Chinese men living in Shanghai was 1.5 per 100,000 while in contrast the rates for Chinese-American men and non-Asian-American men were 15.1 and 48.1 per 100,000, respectively. The wide incidence gap appears related to dietary rather than genetic factors.

Recent studies of low prostate cancer mortality in Japanese men not only link with a low-fat diet but also a diet high in soy product content typical of Japanese men. These favorable findings caused a 1991 National Cancer Institute (NCI) workshop to recommend soy products rather than isolated compounds because soybeans contain several potential anticarcinogens that may work together to suppress the invasion and spread of prostate cancer. The May 1997 *Mayo Clinic Health Letter* points out that "some researchers suggest that substances in soy may cause changes at the cellular level that hinder cancer cell growth." Cohort studies of 14,000 Adventist men found that increasing consumption of beans, lentils, peas, tomatos, raisins, dates, and dried fruit significantly decreased risk for prostate cancer.

Tofu may not be the first thing a man chooses from an oriental restaurant menu, but soy milk poured over breakfast cereal or tofu salad instead of egg salad are healthful ways to get the taste without the negative effects. Tofu can also be used to make puddings and cheesecake or as a substitute for cheese in lasagna. Soy products contain phytoestrogens, which may help ward off prostate cancer. Soy's strongest prostate cancer–fighting compound is genistein, which blocks the formation of blood vessels around new tumors, freezing their growth. The Japanese consume about 20 to 80 mg of genistein daily; Americans consume only 1 to 3 mg. Early research points to genistein as the likely reason that the incidence of prostate cancer among Japanese men is about 35% lower than the incidence in American men.

Hot flashes are virtually unknown among middle-aged women in Japan. My dear wife, Cynthia, was recently diagnosed with a type of breast cancer determined to be hormone receptive. She was immediately removed from estrogen therapy and her hot flashes returned. According to a bimonthly publication from US TOO!, International Inc., which discussed the properties of genistein, estrogens in soy are believed to act like hormone replacement therapy to prevent hot flash irritation without the risks associated with actual hormone therapy. Cynthia tried four tablets of genistein (15 mg each) per day and within the first 24 hours her hot flash symptoms disappeared. One evening, she forgot to take her genistein tablets and the hot flashes returned—certainly strong anecdotal evidence.

On another front, I always preferred my steak or burger charred on the outside. I ordered the end cut of the prime rib. Despite being one of summer's most tasty pleasures, barbecuing meat or fish improperly may create two kinds of chemicals that can cause genetic mutations that result in cancer. In a 1996 study the NCI found people who usually ate their beef well done had more than triple the stomach cancer risk as people who ate meat medium rare. Other studies found diets heavy in well done, fried, or barbecued meats may boost risk of colorectal and, perhaps pancreatic or breast cancer. Human and animal studies taken together offer compelling, if not conclusive, evidence.

Does this mean the pleasures of outdoor cooking must be sacrificed? No, it means that cooking techniques must be updated! The most obvious are to lower cooking temperatures, precook meat in a microwave, or wrap meat in foil before placing it over that open flame. "I think we know these compounds are likely human carcinogens," says Dr. Nancy Snyderwine, NCI's top chemical carcinogenesist. What needs to be avoided is cooking at high temperatures, creating a billowing flame, and having fat drip down and burn, which emits a flavorful aroma, but potentially unhealthy result. This is the process that coats the food with carcinogens, which are formed when the fat drips down into the open flame. There's that fat connection again! "That's what you really want to avoid," says Dr. Snyderwine.

John Weisburger, former director of the AHF facility at Valhalla, New York, has suggested that some marinades used to coat meats could block the formation of carcinogens. "Until then, think of the grill as providing a brief finishing touch to glaze your food, not to torch it," notes Weisburger.

"If every once in a while you want to eat forbidden food, it's OK, as long as it's not a regular habit," says Moshe Shike, Director of Clinical Nutrition at Memorial Sloan-Kettering Cancer Center in New York. "Amid a diet rich in fruits and vegetables containing natural cancer-fighting compounds, " he says, "an occasional barbecue isn't harmful." It may be easier to view this as "putting on sunscreen" before you go out to play.

Finally, a recent dietary finding from Harvard University raised an eyebrow, as well as a smile or two. A study of 48,000 men showed that those who consumed the most lycopene, a powerful antioxidant found in abundance in tomato products, had a 21% lower risk of prostate cancer. Those men who had two to four servings a week of tomato sauce had a 34% lower risk, and even two to four servings a week of pizza reduced the risk by 15%.

According to John Erdman, Ph.D., Director of the Nutritional Sciences Division at the University of Illinois, Urbana, fat helps move lycopene into the blood stream, so pizza and pasta are smarter choices. "Just remember—you don't need triple cheese or double meat on that large pie," warned Erdman. "You don't need a large pie," Cynthia reminds me.

Yes, my first reaction was "who, me?" But this comes down to a direct cost-benefit analysis. If I enjoy my life now and I want to go on enjoying my life for more years I have to take charge of, among other things, my dietary habits.

The relationship between dietary factors and prostate cancer is complex, making it difficult to separate the effect of a given nutrient from other components of the diet and to identify an association with a given cancer. Overall, however, a higher intake of dietary fat seems to be associated with a higher risk for developing prostate cancer. How dietary fat is related to this higher risk is unclear.

An Alarming Trend Continues

The annual incidence of new prostate cancer cases continues to grow at an alarming rate. In 1992 it was 132,000 cases, in 1994 it hit 200,000, in 1996 the number jumped to a reported 314,500, and in 1997 it is projected that it will reach 344,500, representing 29% of all cancer cases, according to the American Cancer Society. The death statistics for prostate cancer are equally impressive, now estimated to reach 42,000 men in 1997.

When revisiting the growth history of cancer cells it becomes even more clear why early detection remains a patient's best chance for a cure and survival of any form of cancer. Attention to a low-fat diet and avoiding other risk factors may further help improve a man's chances for either slowing the progression of prostate cancer or supplementing aggressive treatment therapy during the clinical stage of the disease.

Scientists at Texas A&M University's Institute of Biosciences and Technology (IBT) in Houston report that their studies suggest that a diet rich in vegetables, fruits, whole grains, and soy could help men avoid prostate cancer, currently the second leading cause of death among men. Although environmental factors such as more pollution and greater consumption of dietary fat in the United States were thought to cause the steady jump in prostate disease, research has yet to prove a connection. IBT turned its attention to defining the active ingredients in foods that keep prostates healthy. By better understanding how food ingredients work in both normal and diseased prostate tissues the researchers intend to work with plant experts to develop new plant strains as foods in the diet, as purified agents in food additives, or as pharmaceuticals used in treatment.

The NCI has an entire research section dedicated to assembling, classifying, and evaluating the medicinal benefits of global plant life. Contractors from around the globe collect and send plant specimens to NCI for laboratory investigation. Currently some 35,000 plant samples, representing between 9000 to 10,000 different species, and over 6000 marine samples have been collected.

Work in progress at the University of Alabama indicates that soybean-derived isoflavones (genistein and daidzein) suppress growth of human prostate cancer cell lines in vitro. Although the data are still preliminary, the tendency is to return to the diet characteristics of Japanese and Chinese men as benchmarks for improved chances of prostate cancer prevention and as an adjunct to prostate cancer treatment.

Filling the Gap in Knowledge

Nutrition has never been a major component in physician training. Of the 125 medical schools in the United States, only 25% require a course in nutrition. The estimated average length of physician training in nutrition during 4 years of medical school is about 2.5 hours.

In 1996 the Division of Cancer Prevention and Control (DCPC) and the Division of Cancer Biology (DCB) of the NCI initiated a request for multidisciplinary nutrition and basic biology research related to the prevention of cancer, with emphasis on breast cancer and prostate cancer. Their goal is to improve the understanding of the roles of dietary patterns, individual dietary constituents, and nutritional status in progression and prevention of cancer and they defined three distinct objectives: (1) to increase the pool of quality applications dealing with nutrition and human cancer prevention, (2) to explain the effects of nutrition on cancer initiation, promotion, progression, and prevention, and (3) to promote transfer of knowledge of the impact of nutrition on the biology of cancer into dietary interventions for its prevention.

Nutrition and Prostate Cancer Patient Trials

Dr. Wynder and Dr. Fair announced in the October 1996 *Journal of Urology* the initiation of a four-part, randomized intervention trial on prostate cancer patients who had previously undergone radical prostatectomy and whose PSA had subsequently become positive. Patients will be separated into four groups with the following dietary regimen:

Group 1   A low-fat diet (15% of calories only)
Group 2   A nutritional cocktail of 200µg selenium, 800 IU vitamin E, and a soy product containing 16 mg genistein
Group 3   A low-fat diet plus nutritional cocktail
Group 4   A control group

Initially, the PSA levels will be compared among members of the intervention groups and the control group. The final end point is to be measured by survival. A similar AHF study is being considered for patients with localized or advanced prostate cancer who elect not to be treated and who are followed up with observation-only protocols or those given radiation treatment. The PSA will be used as a measure of tumor volume and other factors related to local progression and/or circulation of tumor cells.

There seems to be strong empirical evidence that dietary influences impact the promotion-progression stage of the natural history of the disease and therefore mortality. The marked difference in diet and fat consumption among Asian men and American men of Asian descent argues strongly for the potential benefits of *adjuvant diet* treatment for prostate patients, as a *supplement* to aggressive treatment for clinical prostate cancer. "For older men, the dietary effect appears to apply principally for older men (over age 60)" (West DW, Slattery ML, Robinson LM, French TK,Mahoney AW. Adult Dietary Intake and Prostate Cancer Risk in Utah: A Case-Controlled Study With Special emphasis on Aggressive Tumors. *Cancer Causes Control* 2: 85-94, 1991; and Kolonel L, Hankin JH, Yoshizawa CN. Vitamin A and Prostate Cancer in Elderly Men: Enhancement of Risk. *Cancer Research* 47: 2982-2985, 1987).

"While scientists and nutritionists, as well as the lay public, may find it difficult to regard a diet providing only 10% to 15% of calories as fat optimal, as well as achievable in terms of economics and taste, the fact remains that clinical prostate cancer is rare among men on such a diet" (Wynder EL, Rose DP, Cohen LA. Nutrition and Prostate Cancer: A Proposal for Dietary Intervention. *Nutrition and Cancer*, 1994).

The Role of Stress in Prostate Cancer

Like a slow poison, stress compromises good health. Unfortunately, when stress becomes part of the daily routine, the body starts to wear down at an accelerated rate. According to a 1996 Princeton Survey Research Associates poll, over 1000 adults report feeling more stressed than ever before. Of those polled, 65% feel stressed at least one day a week compared with 55% just a decade earlier. Much of what we do today is fast paced as technology follows us beyond the time boundaries of the traditional workday—the laptop computer used in the middle of the night or the ever-present pager now hooked on the belt that beeps on weekdays, evenings, and weekends. I often describe living and working in today's information-rich global economy as living in "dog years," where each year of our lives is equivalent to 7 in an earlier time.

We know that stress can weaken the immune system and in turn damage health. Research indicates that there are indeed relationships between stress and disease and that emotions can influence the course of an illness. During a stress reaction or emotional upheaval, hormone levels increase within the body. When this reaction is not sufficient to cope, the stressor maintains its attack. At this point resistance enters the picture. If stress is not managed, eventually fatigue sets in and the exhaustion stage overwhelms it. This becomes the point at which diseases most likely "creep up" on the body. During this stage depression and anxiety are common, and serious illness, even death, becomes a possibility.

We know that prostate cancer has had 10 or 20 years to evolve before it is detected in most men. We also know that in understanding the growth cycle of the disease the tumor has been actively growing for at least 10 years before it reaches the size of a sugar cube, the dimensions that can first be palpated by a well-trained finger during a digital examination.

The doctor's words "this is an early-stage prostate cancer: or "we're lucky we caught this early" only mean that the patient may be a good candidate for curative treatment, which may help us better understand *why* we and others place such heavy and repeated emphasis on early screening and possible detection.

Wrapping Up

A man's attention to a change in dietary habit and stress reduction may help slow the progress of prostate cancer. And if the absolute relationship between dietary fat intake and the nourishment of cells that progress from in situ to clinical prostate cancer cannot be completely understood, we can be confident that adjusting a man's eating habits to a lower fat diet earlier rather than later cannot hurt and almost certainly may help his overall health. Like early prostate screening, good dietary habits become a win-win proposition.

For the younger man undergoing treatment for prostate cancer or the older man for whom the doctor recommends "watchful waiting" an adjustment to a low-fat diet seems only prudent. After all, a low-fat diet has been found to be helpful in preventing many severe diseases in both men and women. At this stage of clinical research, a man has everything to gain and little to lose (except some unneeded extra weight) by adhering to a lower fat regimen.

In my mind there is little doubt that for 10 years preceding the discovery of my locally advanced prostate cancer I functioned at stress levels too high for good health. For the most part, I followed a less than ideal diet, at least as I presently understand it in relation to prostate cancer. But that is now history.

According to Dr. David Bostwick, a Mayo Clinic pathologist, the only species in the animal kingdom other than a man to develop prostate cancer is the dog. Think for a moment about the typical diet man feeds his best friend.

Patients and their families should use this information as background data of the current state of knowledge or ignorance about nutrition as it relates to prostate cancer to discuss with their physician partner—their treating urologist, oncologist or radiation therapist. Keep in mind, however, that the evidence related to a causal link between dietary fat and prostate cancer is growing. Although still somewhat circumstantial, it is more than anecdotal, it is increasingly compelling evidence.

Chapter 11

For the Woman Who Cares

Women are more realistic about health issues than men, and they are usually much more comfortable talking about health issues. Men, as a rule, may resist undergoing important tests, especially the DRE screening test. A woman can help save a man's life, whether he is her husband, father, brother, son, or close friend, by becoming familiar with some of the typical questions and objections that a man might raise regarding a prostate examination (see p. 153). If the screening results indicate prostate cancer, the woman has just been given an even larger role. Illness or a life-threatening disease is not something a man deals with easily. Many men have been socialized to view illness as a weakness or personal failing, and they resist anything that threatens their sense of control over their bodies, their environment, and their self-appointed roles.

Looking Forward

The key to saving his life is in looking forward. For the woman who cares, there are endless opportunities to notice small changes in his daily habits, such as in urinary frequency—first getting up one or more times at night, then soon afterward, a distinct difference in sound as his urine flow slows.

He will have a ready explanation at first—a plausible excuse. It is not that he means to practice self-delusion; rather, it is a man's natural tendency to attribute changes in bodily function to an "input/output problem," such as too many cups of coffee, more Cokes than usual at his desk, or that one beer that goes through him more quickly than it used to. The man's logic holds that if inputs are modified, outputs will also be altered.

Changes show up in small but insidious ways. The movie at the local cineplex now seems too long to make it to the end. At parties, he feels a need to find the bathroom. During a routine drive, he suddenly is glad to pull off at a rest area, when for years he was "the desert-dry guy."

What do these changes mean? Your local library or bookshop should have one or more books on prostate disease. Contact the American Cancer Society for literature. Call a local urologic clinic and ask for some brochures on prostate disease. Not all symptoms mean prostate cancer; educate yourself about benign prostatic hyperplasia, which is as common in men as they age as is graying hair. However, the incidence of prostate cancer, even in men under age 40, is high enough to warrant your attention. If he is into "testosterone denial," as I like to call it, the time has come for *you* to take charge of the situation.

Find out about the PSA test. Seldom a month goes by that there is not a magazine or newspaper article on PSA screening, written in easy-to-understand terms. This test has proved to be a lifesaver in more than one instance. My own experience is a testament to that fact.

Take the initiative. Make an appointment for him with a competent urologist for a prostate screening examination—a DRE *and* a PSA test. Many community hospitals now offer free or very low cost prostate screening clinics. Watch your local newspaper or call your local hospital for the date and time of the next prostate screening clinic. If the test results prove negative, great! Nothing can beat peace of mind. Mark his calendar for same time, same place, next year. Consider it his annual reunion.

You may have to take a very active part in seeing that he follows through on screening, but his life is worth risking a confrontation or being accused of pushing him. Self-care is an area that many men have neglected for all their adult lives and have gotten by with it, for the most part. He may not, probably will not, tell you how he feels about getting such a screening. Denial overrides reason.

Not long ago, Bob, my life insurance adviser, called to pitch some new program. I brought him up to date with my recent experiences. Since we are about the same age, I asked whether he had recently had a prostate screening examination. After some hemming and hawing, Bob confessed that he had *never in his life* allowed a doctor to administer a DRE. It was simply "objectionable" to him to have a doctor explore his body like that. I told him to go have a screening examination and not to call me back until he had done so. It was not the usual way to get rid of an insurance salesman.

While writing these words, I realized it had been several months since Bob and I had last spoken. He never called back. I stopped typing, picked up the phone, and called to ask him what had happened. Bob reported that he had had a PSA test the week after we first talked and was much relieved to learn it was just 1.8. But he still had not submitted himself to the DRE. After a 30-minute plea on my part, he promised to take that step to safeguard his own life. In closing, I threatened to call his wife, to which he responded that she is worse than he is in tracking her own preventive care. Perhaps that is why Bob is such a strong believer in life insurance.

The woman has a special role. She can observe small changes; she can keep an eye on his physical routine. But it is not easy to help. The prostate is not an easy subject to broach with a man; it has both physical and sexual function overtones. The fear of a catastrophic illness can paralyze the strongest man—and a disease related to a man's sexuality, even more so.

Knowing the truth is the first step. This gives you both a second chance. At an American Cancer Society Prostate Cancer Forum, Laura Phlager, the partner of a prostate cancer survivor, summed it up this way: "The woman is obligated to get involved. Her vantage point allows her good observation. And she must not stop until action has been taken."

What If the Screening Test Results Are Positive?

A diagnosis of prostate cancer is not the end of the world; it is not a death sentence—it is a call to arms!

Reconnaissance has identified the enemy and found its stronghold, and battle lines have been drawn. Together you must both begin to outline the strategic decisions that will guide your campaign against his disease. At times you will be his aide de camp—and sometimes you will have to be the general in his stead.

Not long ago, while waiting to pick up my dog, Cookie, at the veterinarian's office, I got into a conversation with the receptionist. She seemed very distressed and told me of her father, who had recently been diagnosed with prostate cancer but who refused to go for treatment. Based on some deeply held mind-set, he had concluded that what will be will be. I asked if he had ever served in the armed forces and learned that he was a veteran of both World War II and the Korean War. "Tell him this is war," I suggested. "It's either cancer or him. There can be only one winner. There is no truce; there can be no cease-fire."

The man in your life needs you now, more than he ever realized. He needs another set of eyes and ears. Once I learned that my prostate diagnosis was in fact cancer, Cynthia decided to accompany me to all meetings with the consulting urologist. And it was a good thing. We were in this as a team and we would see it through together.

The woman plays a pivotal role in literature research—not so much in gathering data and information as in playing "devil's advocate" to help him avoid coming to a premature conclusion. The nine underlying principles of problem solving (see Chapter 6 and Appendix B) can help you calibrate his focus on the right questions. Together, you can reach the best course of action for him.

At first, his mind may seem to wander, to focus on matters of less consequence than a diagnosis of cancer. "What's going to happen at work?" he wonders. "This couldn't come at a worse moment—it's a bad time to be taking days away from the job." (Is there ever a good time for prostate cancer to show up?) "How am I going to pay for all this?" You can help him remain focused on matters that may save his life.

After each doctor's visit Cynthia and I compared notes. She heard things that I completely missed; she sensed things I did not sense. At a time like this a woman's antennae seem especially sensitive to all kinds of small things. We immediately talked about everything and then went over it several times. The woman who cares needs to keep her man talking about different aspects of the impending decision, not letting him retreat into that shell so often used by men to avoid talking about difficult issues.

Soon enough he will be confronted with the treatment dilemma—and a decision. He needs your help to sort out his feelings and yours. The treatment decision can quickly become enmeshed in considerations that are not always truly relevant to a healthy outcome. He not only needs to talk about *his* feelings but also to hear how *you* are coping. Mayo Clinic pathologist David Bostwick, M.D., calls the patient and his significant other a "unit of care." Now is not the time to drift into separate corners but to come together as a team. Soon you will decide who will be joining your team.

Recently, I received a call from a friend of a friend who had just learned he was a new member of the prostate cancer club. At age 61 he was starting his life over, so to speak; he and his second wife had been married just 6 years. Understandably, his entire focus was on finding a treatment to retain potency. There were many approaches discussed in the literature—nerve-sparing radical prostatectomy, radioactive seed implants, but no procedure offered a clear or guaranteed outcome. "What are your wife's feelings in all of this?" I asked. "She's left it all to me," he sighed. I suggested that they both read Michael Korda's *Man to Man*, a story much like the story he related to me.

Most important is that the man's life is at stake. But is life just your sex life? He needs your support and encouragement and full participation, now more than ever. In addition, both of you need to understand and live with the implications of any chosen course of treatment. The fact is that even the best of surgeons or radiologists do not know what they will find when they go after prostate cancer. Recall that more than 50% of prostate glands removed by the radical prostatectomy procedure have been found on postoperative laboratory examination to have been understaged. In other words, the cancer had progressed farther and faster than had been thought before surgery.

He needs your help to master the situation. He needs to develop a realistic perspective. He needs to order his priorities for the right reasons. It has everything to do with both of you maintaining a positive mind-set throughout this very stressful period.

Work with him toward getting a second opinion. You may both be perfectly comfortable with your diagnosing urologist. But the value in the second opinion comes from learning the new and unexpected rather than merely getting confirmation that prostate cancer is present. Many times the second opinion may cast an entirely different light on the situation and affect the treatment decision. By the time you pursue this step, you will both be much better prepared to engage the physician in a meaningful, productive conversation.

"In Treatment and in Healing"

Maybe the marriage vow should be a little more explicit. We seldom give much thought when we marry to what "in sickness and in health" may truly mean within the marital partnership. After an event such as a diagnosis of prostate cancer, suddenly that vow represents a real commitment of caring. There is much to be done after the prostate treatment also. Whatever treatment is selected, he is not going to be in shape to do much around the house for a while (assuming he did something before).

Get some outside help. Cynthia insisted she could do it all herself. Although she tried valiantly, it just was not possible. The house seems twice its size when there is no one to help clean it. The yard seems to grow weeds faster when there is only one person to attend to it. Even the appointed hour to take out the dog comes around more quickly. There is less time to do the same things.

Find someone to help with routine chores—grocery shopping, transportation. It is not forever; more like a few weeks until his recovery process stabilizes a bit. When friends and neighbors say, "If there's anything I can do, just call me," *take them up on it.* Someday they may need the favor returned. And if you are also carrying a full-time job during all of this (as Cynthia was), it is best to just be direct with your boss. You may receive some support from an unanticipated direction.

Many insurance carriers cover in-home caregiver services. It is surprising how just a little assistance can go a long way in helping you both heal. Don't be shy. There are lots of extra surprises waiting for you during the healing period.

Watch him closely for any signs of depression. Get him to talk about his feelings. He may exhibit signs of melancholia; it is a natural by-product of two new realities—his loss of libido and his deep sense of lost innocence. He is no longer young, virile, invincible, immortal. This is a true paradigm shift—a new view of the world. Guiding him from the outset toward help from a psychologist, psychiatrist, or licensed professional counselor can help forestall greater complications later.

There are many adjustments for you both during the healing process. It is a time when staying "in touch" with one another is vital. The old rules that previously governed family communications are habits formed over years that may need to be reevaluated in light of new realities.

Home Nursing

The woman carries the bulk of the load during healing, even though she is not the patient. In an era of managed health care plans, it is not unusual to have the patient come home from the hospital still requiring close attention from a caregiver.

Home postoperative care often includes urine collection bags, with their attendant connecting tubes, which need to be changed for nighttime. These tubes are simple to manipulate but need to be sterile and airtight. They can prove challenging to change for someone new to home nursing. And there are always a few bandages that need replacement. Make certain you have an adequate supply of all necessary equipment when you leave the hospital.

The woman needs to ask the doctor and nurses at the hospital to carefully and slowly demonstrate the steps she will have to take alone when she will be wrestling this paraphernalia at home. This is a difficult time for the woman to take on-the-job nurse's training. The man may not feel much like helping, at least not in the beginning.

Even taking a shower will probably be harder for him to handle alone, especially in a weakened condition. And unexpected occurrences are almost certain to surface. If so, don't be afraid to phone the doctor or nurse designate, day or night, to check it out. Is what he is experiencing to be expected? Can his discomfort be relieved in some way? Bladder spasms, for instance, can be very painful and distressing. When in doubt—call and ask. It can help prevent other problems later. This is not the time for reticence; it is your health care team and you have every right to call for help when you need it.

It is always tougher to be on the outside of the pain. Both of you have been stricken and now are fighting back together against prostate cancer. Recovery from prostate cancer involves more than healing the body—you will need to replenish your exhausted emotional resources as well. Both of you must be kind to your *selves* and to each other. You are also in a better position than anyone else to treat your partner as a whole person, not merely as a patient or invalid. Conscious and constant insistence on maintaining this "whole and well" mental image is an essential factor in carrying him toward recovery.

Strategies for More Effective Communication*

- **Use "I" statements rather than "you" statements.** For example, "I sometimes feel you're too busy to listen to me," instead of "You never listen to what I'm telling you."
- **Make a direct statement to express your needs,** instead of asking indirect questions. For example, "I'd like something to eat," instead of "Are you hungry?"
- **Don't expect your partner to be a mind-reader.**
- **Avoid "gunnysacking"**—the habit of stuffing all your past conflicts into an imaginary bag and dragging them all out during an argument, whether they are relevant or not.
- **Reduce the emotional level of your exchanges.** Avoid anger, sarcasm, threats, yelling—all roadblocks to healthy and productive communication.

*From Bostwick D, MacLennan G, Larson T. The American Cancer Society. Prostate Cancer: What Every Man—and His Family—Needs to Know. New York: Villard Books, 1996.

Tackling His Action-Blocking Excuses

Here are some of the excuses he may offer initially for avoiding screening tests, along with some examples of how you might go about removing those blocks.

"Prostate problems are an old man's problem."
- False. Prostate problems can hit any man, especially after age 40.
- If there is a family history of prostate cancer, that is even more of a reason for concern.

"Why waste the money? I don't feel like anything is wrong."
- Go anyway. They call prostate cancer the "silent killer" for a good reason. Each year more than 40,000 American men die of prostate cancer because their condition was diagnosed too late for treatment.
- There are usually no symptoms (or only very subtle ones) of prostate disease in the early stages. And that is when prostate cancer is most curable!

- If you wait until you develop serious symptoms, it may be too late to cure the cancer.

"I don't like the idea of some doctor putting his finger up my backside (the DRE)."

- Most men don't like it. But the prostate is an internal organ that cannot be looked at directly.
- Women's reproductive organs are internal, and women are more used to submitting their bodies to a yearly internal examination. Are women really more brave than men?
- It may seem somewhat awkward, but the safeguard is worth it.

"I heard this DRE thing is uncomfortable."

- The examination is simple and quick. It's over before you realize it.
- What are a few seconds of mild discomfort compared with possibly saving your life?
- An annual mammogram is uncomfortable also and takes a lot longer.

"During my last checkup the doctor didn't poke around my prostate."

- Because some men balk at prostate examinations, not all doctors do them routinely.
- Every man over 40 needs to ask for a DRE and the simple PSA blood test.

"I'm too busy right now to go for a checkup."

- I'll make the appointment for you. I'll even pick you up at work and drive you to the doctor's office.
- Catching problems early takes less time from your busy schedule than treating a serious illness would.
- If the Chairman of the Board of Intel can find the time, so can you.

"If I have a prostate problem, it means the end of my sex life."

- This is not true. There is sex after prostate treatment!
- In fact, the earlier you catch it, the better the chance of its not affecting your sex life.

"If something is wrong with my prostate, I would rather not know. Prostate cancer is incurable."

- General Norman Schwarzkopf said, "It's stupid for any man to die of this disease." And his prostate cancer was detected by DRE.

- If caught early, many prostate cancers are curable.
- The odds are stacked against treating and curing an advanced case of prostate cancer. So there is every reason to have an early—and regular—prostate examination.
- If the disease is not caught until too late for treatment, it is a very painful way to die.

If signs of a prostate problem are present, encourage him to get prompt professional help. By expressing your support and sharing your knowledge of prostate problems, your actions can help reduce the stress and the feelings of isolation that the man may experience during the screening, diagnosis, treatment, and healing processes.

Ultimately he will love you for it.

◆
_____

Afterword

Michael J. Wehle, M.D.

When Allen Salowe asked me to write an afterword for this book, I was flattered and pleased to contribute to his worthwhile endeavor. I thought writing an essay on prostate cancer would be a relatively easy task, since I encounter some aspect of prostate cancer almost every day of my life. Why, then, was it so difficult to write this afterword?

I wanted the essay to be clear and helpful, so the reader could better understand prostate cancer. However, the subject of prostate cancer is anything but clear. Urologists often feel frustrated and inadequate as they try to present an honest appraisal of the treatment options to each patient newly diagnosed with prostate cancer. The patient wants a definitive answer about what treatment is best for him, but that black-and-white solution often does not exist. Frequently, I feel the patient and his family leave my presence in a more discouraged and confused state than when they first came to hear what I had to say.

Unfortunately, there is an abundance of conflicting data concerning prostate cancer, making it all the more confusing to the patient and physician. It is also difficult not to project one's own bias onto the patient. The urologist is a surgeon and sees things through a surgeon's eyes. A radiotherapist is a radiotherapist and has a bias toward radiation therapy. I think most urologists and radiotherapists try to evaluate the data in an honest and fair way. As a urologist I often realize that surgery is not for everyone, and some patients are better served by other forms of treatment, such as radiation therapy. In certain instances and situations, I do not always know what to recommend as the best treatment for a patient with localized prostate cancer. Recognizing this makes me uncomfortable.

On the other hand, it would be false to say that there is no good information to help patients and physicians select the appropriate treatment. A plethora of excellent scientific data exists to help us make a sound choice. The challenge for urologists is to understand and assimilate these data and be able to clearly and honestly communicate it to our patients.

I hope to present some of the salient data regarding prostate cancer to help the patient and his family better understand the disease and make the treatment choice that best serves his needs. For optimal results, it is important that the patient understand his treatment—and believe in it. It is vital that the patient and family involve themselves in this treatment and feel confidence in their therapy and the abilities of their physicians. To achieve this level of comfort, the patient must first understand and ultimately accept his disease. By becoming an active partner in his treatment and trying to understand about prostate cancer, he will have taken the very first and most important step to recovery.

The Facts

Approximately 317,000 Americans were newly diagnosed in 1996 with prostate cancer. Of these men, more than 60% had an early (localized) form of the disease. The other 40% had a more advanced form of prostate cancer at the time of diagnosis. The detection of prostate cancer has increased enormously. In 1993, 164,000 American men were newly diagnosed.[1]

A man in the United States has approximately a 10% life-time risk of developing prostate cancer. Approximately every 3 minutes, one man is diagnosed with prostate cancer in the United States. The number of patients dying from prostate cancer is second only to lung cancer. Approximately 40,000 men a year will die of prostate cancer in this country; it is responsible for approximately 3 of every 100 deaths among American men. Unfortunately, the death toll from prostate cancer has been increasing steadily. Approximately 20% of the patients who develop *clinically significant* prostate cancer will die from their disease.[1]

Risk Factors

Unfortunately, we do not know the cause of prostate cancer, and the means for preventing prostate cancer are not clearly understood. We have, however, learned that certain groups of men are at increased risk for developing the disease. African-Americans seem to have a higher incidence of prostate cancer. Northern Europeans also seem to have a high incidence of the disease, whereas Asians have a relatively low incidence.[2,3] It is difficult to determine the reasons for these differences. It is probable that environment, diet, and genetic influences are factors. Some data show that patients with a high-fat diet are at increased risk. Certainly, if a patient has a first-degree relative or relatives who have developed prostate cancer, the likelihood of his developing prostate cancer may be as much as 5 to 10 times higher.[2,3] The frequency of sexual activity, the presence of prostatitis, benign prostatic hyperplasia, a history of smoking, or activity level do not appear to influence the development of prostate cancer to any great degree.

Testosterone, the principal androgenic male hormone, must be present for prostate cancer to develop and thrive. Prostate cancer is almost nonexistent among patients who had low or undetectable testosterone levels before puberty. Testosterone, when given to laboratory rats, causes an increase in the development of prostate cancer. The removal of testosterone by either surgical or chemical castration will cause most prostate cancer to regress for a period of time.[4,5]

Age appears to be a risk factor. Certainly, the older a man gets, the more likely he is to develop prostate cancer. Autopsy studies indicate a high percentage of histologic prostate cancer (that is, detected microscopically) as men become older. These studies show that approximately 30% of the men examined over the age of 50 have histologic prostate cancer present. In an 80-year-old man, the likelihood is 70% to 80% that he will have histologic prostate cancer.[6]

Vasectomy has been considered as a possible risk factor. Much attention was given to this several years ago, based on a Dartmouth study that indicated that there may be increased risk of prostate cancer in men who have had a vasectomy for 10 years or longer.[7,8] Obviously, this finding was disturbing to many men who had undergone vasectomy. However, when these data were analyzed more closely, it became apparent that the increased risk of developing prostate cancer from vasectomy was very weak. The National Institutes of Health also analyzed the data; they thought that there was an increased risk as a result of detection bias only. It was their conclusion that vasectomy is unlikely to be a major risk factor for developing prostate cancer.[9]

Confusion

Considerable confusion exists regarding the natural history of prostate cancer. Many think that prostate cancer is a relatively benign disease and that most men die *with* their cancer, not *from* it. On the other hand, the 41,400 American men who will die of prostate cancer this year might find that to be understated. Which are we to believe? Are there two kinds of prostate cancer, one that seems to behave in a clinically benign way and one that will progress and kill?

Using the numbers regarding the presence of histologic prostate cancer and the fact that there are 30 million men in the United States over the age of 50, we can conclude that 10 million men in the United States have prostate cancer now. As I noted earlier, 300,000 men were newly diagnosed with prostate cancer in 1996. This would be a small fraction of the projected 10 million men who are thought to harbor prostate cancer based on data from autopsy series. These facts enlighten us to several important points. First, our current ability to detect small, *clinically insignificant* prostate cancer is inadequate. Second, not all patients with prostate cancer have a cancer that is clinically important. These cancers would not necessarily demand detection and treatment. Finally, it underscores the point that we must comprehend the natural history of prostate cancer to better appreciate the significance of prostate cancer present in each patient. We need to understand the natural history of the disease to determine whether to treat or not to treat a patient with prostate cancer. Understanding the natural history helps gain insight as to which treatment is appropriate for a particular individual.

Natural History

We know that in the early form of most prostate cancers the cells have a tendency to divide slowly. It is estimated from work done at Stanford University that the *doubling time* (the time it takes for cancer cells to double in number) of a typical prostate cancer cell is about 2 to 4 years.[10] As the cell volume increases, the degree of cellular differentiation begins to change. As the cell becomes *less differentiated* (less like normal prostate cells), it has the tendency to become more aggressive (apt to metastasize) and to have a shorter doubling time. Pathologists think a tumor volume of approximately 0.5 cc to 1 cc is significant. It is at this volume—approximately the size of a small sugar cube—that the tumor has a tendency to escape the confines of the prostate, and the cells have a tendency to become less differentiated. Ironically, it is also at this volume that an examiner would be able to palpate a tumor by DRE. Thus by the time the tumor reaches a volume that can be palpated, the cells have started to become less differentiated and the tumor has likely spread beyond the confines of the gland. It is important to keep in mind that currently we have no way to eradicate prostate cancer once it has spread beyond the prostate. Based on a doubling time of approximately 2 years, the cancer may have been present for as long as 10 years before it has grown to a volume that will become harmful to the patient. Using DRE as the only means of detection for early prostate cancer would not allow us to detect cancer in many of our patients in the early localized form.[11]

In studies in which the prostate gland was removed in patients who were thought (based on DRE findings) to have disease confined to the prostate, only 50% of these patients actually had confined disease. The other 50% had already exhibited metastasis of the cancer. These studies indicate that in diagnosis by DRE, there is a tendency to underestimate the amount of disease present.[12,13] Logic suggests that if we could detect prostate cancer in an earlier form, perhaps we could reduce the mortality of the disease.

Early Detection

We know from our experience with other cancers that early detection can improve survival and decrease the morbidity of the disease. No proof currently exists, however, that indicates that early detection of prostate cancer will decrease the number of patients dying from the disease. It may be years before these data are gathered, but even skeptics have to admit that just because the data are currently not available does not imply that the hypothesis is not true. Based on current clinical data, urologists recommend the DRE and PSA evaluation for men over the age of 50 who are interested in detecting early prostate cancer. If the patient has a family history of the disease or is an African-American, age 40 is recommended as a time to begin methods for early detection. If the PSA test or DRE yields abnormal results, a transrectal ultrasound evaluation and biopsy are recommended. Transrectal ultrasound of the prostate when the PSA level or DRE findings are normal has been shown to be ineffective. The use of this detection schema has allowed us to detect a greater number of patients with a localized form of prostate cancer than previous studies in which DRE alone was utilized.[14,15]

PSA Blood Testing

The development and use of the PSA screening test has radically advanced our understanding of prostate cancer. PSA is a proteolytic enzyme secreted by prostate epithelial cells. Normally very small amounts of PSA enter the bloodstream. When the architecture of the prostate is altered, PSA may then enter the circulatory system in larger amounts and be detected in higher levels in the serum. Prostate cancer, prostate inflammation, and benign prostatic hyperplasia are the most common reasons for an elevated PSA level. Other factors such as prostate surgery, biopsy, manipulation, and recent ejaculation may mildly elevate the PSA. PSA has been shown to be more sensitive than DRE in detecting prostate cancer. However, it appears that by using both DRE and PSA, we are better able to detect prostate cancer than by using either method alone.[14-16]

Early detection studies indicate that a range of 0 to 4 nanograms per milliliter (ng/ml) of PSA is a normal standard for most men.[17] Other studies have demonstrated that the PSA level increases with age.[16-18] This is probably because as one becomes older, the architecture of the gland changes as a result of benign prostatic hyperplasia and inflammation. For this reason, an age-adjusted PSA norm was developed. The hope was that by correcting the normal values for younger and older patients, a more accurate PSA method of detecting prostate cancer could be devised. In younger men (between the ages of 40 and 49), a normal range of 0 to 2.5 ng/ml was suggested and in patients of the older age group (70 to 79), a normal range was 0 to 6.5 ng/ml. It was hoped that this would decrease the number of unnecessary biopsies performed on older patients and allow PSA to increase the sensitivity mechanism for detecting earlier prostate cancer in the younger group of patients.[16-18]

PSA can also be used in helping to stage or to estimate the extent of prostate cancer present. The higher the PSA value, the more likely the tumor has escaped the confines of the gland and spread to the lymph nodes or bone. PSA tests also indicate the response to treatment. After a radical prostatectomy (complete removal of the prostate), the PSA value should fall to near zero or the undetectable range. If the value does not fall to an undetectable range or if the PSA increases over time, this indicates the presence of residual disease. We also expect to see a fall in PSA in patients who have undergone radiation therapy. The PSA should then reach a stable plateau. Again, if there is an increase in the PSA level, this could indicate that the tumor has not been eradicated by radiation therapy or that metastatic disease may be present.

The Down Side to PSA

As remarkable a tumor marker as PSA is, it has some shortcomings. It must be realized that as many as 3 of 10 patients who have significant prostate cancer may have a normal PSA value, and some very poorly differentiated tumors have a tendency not to produce PSA. The PSA value may vary by as much as 30% of its value from day to day.[16,19] Finally, other pathologic conditions not associated with prostate cancer may cause a rise in PSA. As many as 20% of patients who have benign prostatic hyperplasia may have an elevated PSA, in the range of 4 to 10 ng/ml. Because of these shortcomings, several variations in the way PSA is measured have been attempted to increase the accuracy and usefulness of the PSA blood test.[20]

PSA Variations
PSA Density

PSA density measures the relation between PSA level and the size and weight of the prostate gland. Prostate gland volume can be determined by transrectal ultrasound. The PSA density helps the physician determine whether the PSA is elevated as a result of prostatic enlargement from benign prostatic hyperplasia or whether it is likely to be caused by prostate cancer. Several studies have shown this to be useful, whereas others have suggested that its usefulness is no more than that of PSA alone.[16,21]

PSA Velocity

PSA velocity is a measurement or change of PSA over time. Often the change in PSA can be more predictive in the presence of prostate cancer than the actual value of PSA.[16] The problem with PSA velocity is that the length of time needed to make PSA velocities useful and accurate has not yet been clearly defined. It is currently recommended that three PSA values be taken at 12-month intervals.

Free and Total PSA

Measuring free and total PSA may be helpful in determining whether a patient's PSA is elevated because of benign disease or is secondary to prostate cancer. Most PSA appears in the blood either attached to another protein (bound) or in a free form with no attached protein (unbound). It appears that the patients who have prostate cancer have a higher percentage of bound PSA. Therefore new tests to measure the amount of bound and unbound PSA may be helpful in detecting early prostate cancer and helping to distinguish prostate cancer from benign prostatic disease.[16,22]

Biopsy

To definitively diagnose prostate cancer, a tissue sample from the prostate is necessary. On occasion, prostate cancer is diagnosed when examining the tissue removed during a transurethral resection of the prostate (TURP). A TURP is performed for benign prostatic disease in most instances, but in 5% to 10% of the cases, cancer is detected in the tissue removed.[23]

Currently, biopsies of the prostate are performed in the office with local anesthesia. Transrectal ultrasound is used to guide the needle exactly to the area of the prostate to be biopsied. A spring-loaded gun shoots the small-gauge needle into the prostate, removing a small sliver of the prostate for pathologic examination. The procedure is not comfortable, but few patients complain that it is painful. Six biopsies are usually taken—from the base, the midportion of the prostate, and the apex from both the left and right sides of the gland.

As in all invasive procedures, there is some risk. There is a 2% risk that bleeding will occur. Patients should be advised not to take aspirin or other medications with anticoagulant properties for an appropriate amount of time preceding the biopsy. A very low incidence of infection can be expected. Antibiotics can be given orally before and after the procedure for maximum protection. It does not appear that a biopsy will cause spread of the cancer or dysfunction of the prostate.

Biopsies of the prostate are also performed after certain prostate cancer treatments, such as cryotherapy (also called cryoablation), external beam radiation, and brachytherapy (placement of radioactive seeds into the prostate tissue). To determine whether all the cancer has been eradicated, the tissue obtained from the prostate is then submitted to the pathologist for microscopic examination.

Grading and Staging
Grading

The grading of a tumor is the pathologist's assessment of how the cells appear in terms of cellular features and the architecture of the tissue as viewed under a microscope. The Gleason grading system looks at the two most prominent areas of the tumor represented on the specimen. The pathologist then assigns a score from 1 to 5. A Gleason score of 1 represents a pattern that does not look all that different from normal cells, with the cells appearing to be well differentiated. A Gleason score of 5 represents poorly differentiated cells; these cells appear very aggressive and very different from normal prostate cells. The scores for the two most prominent areas are then added to give a combined Gleason score. A well-differentiated tumor has a Gleason score of 2 to 4. A moderately differentiated tumor is 5 to 7, and a poorly differentiated tumor is from 8 to 10.[24]

This score is useful for its predictive and prognostic value concerning how the tumor will progress. For example, a patient with a Gleason score of 4 is more likely to do well with any type of prostate cancer treatment, compared with a patient with a Gleason score of 8.[24] The volume of the tumor present in the biopsy also gives the physician an idea of the extent of tumor. The Gleason score is helpful in predicting the likelihood that cancer will spread to the lymph nodes preoperatively. A patient with a Gleason score of 9 has an increased likelihood of having positive lymph nodes. For this reason, the patient may not be a good candidate for a radical retropubic prostatectomy.

Prostate biopsies can underestimate the amount of tumor (sampling error) and potentially miss areas of prostate cancer (false negative). The likelihood of detecting clinically insignificant cancers is very small, since biopsies are taken in only a few of the areas of the prostate. In other words, a sufficient volume of cancer needs to be present for the pathologist to be able to detect the cancer with the tissue from six biopsy sites.

Staging

The stage of prostate cancer is related to the extent of the disease extension. The tumor-node-metastasis (TNM) staging system is the method most commonly used today. Stages T1 and T2 indicate the cancer is confined to the prostate. Stages T3 and T4 suggest local extension of the cancer to surrounding tissues outside the prostate. The N in the staging system indicates whether the cancer involves the surrounding lymph nodes, and the M represents the degree of spread to distant areas of the body. Another staging system, used less often today, is the Whitmore-Jewett (ABCD) system, in which A is related to cancers confined to the prostate found on TURP, B indicates tumors that are palpable but still confined to the prostate, C is a tumor that has extended outside the prostate into surrounding tissue, and D is a tumor that has metastasized into lymph nodes or into bone.

The staging of the tumor can be of two types: *clinical* and *pathologic*. Clinical staging is based on DRE, PSA test results, and radiologic studies such as bone scan or CT scan. Pathologic staging is the actual extent of the disease as seen microscopically by a pathologist. Pathologic staging is the more accurate of the two systems. The pathologic stage can be obtained only when the patient has surgery; therefore patients who undergo radiation therapy but have no tissue removed would not have pathologic staging. Clinical stage often underestimates the extent of the disease by as much as 20% to 25% of the time; it can also overestimate as much as 5% to 10% of the time.

Radiologic studies such as bone scans, abdominal and pelvic CT scans, and magnetic resonance imaging (MRI) can be used to stage patients' tumors. The bone scan is the most commonly used radiologic test for prostate cancer staging. Recently, it has been questioned whether a bone scan is necessary in patients who have low- to moderate-grade tumors, no skeletal symptoms, and a PSA level under 10 ng/ml.[16] The likelihood of a patient having skeletal metastasis is so small that a bone scan may not be necessary. CT scans and MRI studies are used less frequently and only in special circumstances.

Decision Time

Once the appropriate data have been gathered, the physician and the patient should review and discuss the meaning and importance of the test results. It is usually at this time that the reality of having prostate cancer becomes apparent to the patient and his family. A patient with an apparent localized disease is presented with several treatment options; those with more advanced disease have fewer treatments from which to choose. The decision process can be very difficult and confusing. Patients who take an active role in learning as much as they can about their particular cancer seem to have less trouble making their decision. At some point a strong inner voice emerges within the patient to help direct him to the right treatment.

A well-informed physician discusses openly and honestly the pros and cons of all treatment options with as little bias as possible. Every patient is a unique individual, and no one treatment will fit all. In addition to the data germane to the tumor, the patient's age, health, sexual activity, occupation, and finally the patient's inner hopes and fears must be considered. It is my belief that in most instances, given appropriate information, patients choose the treatment option best suited for their particular situation and lifestyle.

Treatments

Time and space do not permit a detailed description of each treatment; these details can be found in a variety of excellent sources. The most important detailed information regarding the treatment options should come from the patient's chosen medical team.

Treatment options can be categorized into one of two groups: (1) curative treatments for localized prostate cancer and (2) palliative treatments for nonlocalized prostate cancer (advanced disease). The current conventional treatments for localized cancer are radical prostatectomy, either by the retropubic approach or the perineal approach, radiation therapy (external beam radiation), and watchful waiting. Treatments currently considered investigational are cryoablation of the prostate and brachytherapy (placement of a radioactive seed into the prostate).

Androgen ablation therapy, or removal of testosterone by either chemical or surgical castration, is the mainstay for advanced prostate cancer. This therapy can be used before definitive treatment in an attempt to decrease the tumor size and the extent of its spread. Currently, it is unknown whether this neoadjuvant treatment has any long-lasting benefit or will improve long-term cancer-free survival. Chemotherapy, unfortunately, has not been found successful in the treatment of metastastic prostate cancer. Radiation therapy can also be initiated for palliative relief from painful bony metastases.

Prostatectomy

Each treatment for localized prostate cancer has advantages and disadvantages. Radical prostatectomy has been performed since the turn of the century. We know that if the cancer is truly localized to the prostate (T1 or T2), radical prostatectomy can provide a life-long disease-free status.[25,26] Cancer-free survival with radical prostatectomy can be expected in 70% to 80% of patients 10 years after initiation of the treatment. Recurrence at the operative site after radical prostatectomy occurs in 8% to 10% of cases.[25,26]

Advances in the technique of radical prostatectomy developed by Walsh et al.[27] in the mid-1980s greatly lowered the morbidity and mortality associated with the procedure. It also allowed preservation of the neurovascular bundles that run along the posterolateral aspect of the prostate. Preservation of these structures allowed improved potency rates after the surgery. Before this development, 100% of patients were impotent after radical prostatectomy. Most urologists think the procedure should be reserved for men who have apparent localized disease, a 10- to 15-year life expectancy, and have good surgical risk factors. In medical centers where the procedure is performed frequently, the complication rates are relatively low. Severe incontinence occurs in approximately 3% to 5% of patients, although mild stress incontinence may occur in 25%. Transfusion is needed in less than 10% of the patients. Mortality associated with the operation is less than 1%. The ability to preserve potency can be as high as 70%.

Patients who are younger with a low-volume form of the disease can expect to have higher rates of potency postoperatively than older patients or those with more extensive disease.[28,29]

A drawback to prostatectomy is that it requires hospitalization (3 to 5 days) and 6 to 8 weeks of convalescence. In addition, the operation is not successful in eradicating the cancer if the disease has extended to tissue surrounding the prostate. Accurate clinical staging of the disease, that is, knowing that the disease is confined to the prostate only, is difficult with our present preoperative testing. Understaging of the cancer can occur in up to 25% of the patients who undergo the surgery.

Radiation Therapy

External beam radiation therapy can be employed to eradicate localized prostate cancer. It is administered with high-dose linear accelerators. The full treatment dose must be given in fractions. With advances in the delivery system and improved radiologic imaging, the potential adverse side effects from external beam radiation therapy have been reduced. A period of 6 to 8 weeks is needed to administer the total treatment. An advantage of radiation therapy is that the treatment can be administered as an outpatient and thus hospitalization is not necessary. Typical side effects include transient diarrhea, uncomfortable voiding, and skin irritation. Some patients can develop severe and chronic bladder and bowel irritation. Incontinence occurs from 1% to 5% of the time, and impotence occurs in at least 50% of the patients.[30]

The greatest drawback to radiation therapy is its inability to totally eradicate the cancer. In at least 40% of the patients who receive radiation for localized prostate cancer, the disease is still present after radiation therapy. Published long-term disease-free survival rates for external beam radiation therapy are impressive, with 15-year data showing a 60% to 70% disease-free survival.[30,31] However, these data were taken before the era of PSA blood test screening. We now know that PSA is a very good and sensitive indicator of persistent disease. A rise in PSA 18 months after external beam radiation strongly indicates residual disease, and in less than 50% of the patients with localized disease treated with radiation do we see a stable PSA.[30] Less than

10% of these patients ever achieve an undetectable level of PSA. Prostate cancer apparently has a clone of cells that are radioresistant.

Brachytherapy is a different form of radiation therapy. It is the placement of radioactive seeds into the prostate through small needles placed through the perineal skin. Most frequently, iodine-125 (^{125}I) seeds are employed. Ultrasonography allows direct vision and accurate placement of each seed. The procedure requires anesthesia and hospitalization. Current data using ^{125}I look promising, but the follow-up period is limited so far. Thus it is difficult to determine whether the treatment is as effective as radical prostatectomy or external beam radiation therapy. Previous clinical studies using brachytherapy showed a 10-year progression-free survival of only 44%.[22,30] It remains to be seen whether the current technique of employing brachytherapy will offer any improved results or will repeat results seen in the past using brachytherapy.

In summary, radical prostatectomy is usually recommended for younger men (under age 75) who are proved to be in good health and have a life expectancy of 10 to 15 years, have localized prostate cancer, and are at low operative risk. Radiation treatment is recommended to patients who are older and have more extensive localized disease or those patients who appear to be a poor surgical risk.

Watchful Waiting

Several recent studies have suggested that watchful waiting is an effective if not superior approach when compared with the more aggressive treatments for localized prostate cancer. Unfortunately, many of these studies have serious flaws, leading to inaccurate conclusions.

It has long been the practice of physicians in this country to recommend watchful waiting as a treatment option to older patients with low-grade, low-stage prostate cancer.[32] We realize from understanding the natural history of the disease that well-differentiated, small-volume tumors take many years of growth before they can be clinically harmful to the patient. Scandinavian studies show that even when patients have tumors of low grade, more than 50% of the patients show progression of their tumor within a 10-year period if the watchful waiting approach is selected. Ultimately 60% of the patients who are diagnosed with cancer at age 70 die of their disease if watchful waiting is employed.[22] If the prostate cancer was discovered at age 55 or younger, 100% of the patients in this study died of prostate cancer if watchful waiting was initiated as the treatment.[22,33] Many men find it psychologically difficult to employ watchful waiting knowing that a growing (albeit slow-growing) cancer is present.

Cryosurgery

Not all patients are comfortable with any of the treatment options discussed previously. All of the options for localized disease have disadvantages, and for these reasons it seems logical to strive to find an effective, less-invasive form of treatment for localized prostate cancer. It is hoped by many that cryotherapy might represent such treatment. Improvements in technique and advances in technology allowed cryotherapy to be reintroduced. Work done by Onik[34] and Cohen in the early 1990s initiated much excitement and wonderment about cryotherapy.

The procedure is performed through five small puncture wounds through the skin. Five small probes are placed in the prostate through these puncture wounds under the guidance of transrectal ultrasound so that the probes are accurately placed in the prostate tissue. A warming catheter is placed through the urethra to keep the urethra warm during the freezing process. Freezing of the prostatic urethral area can cause excess shedding of devitalized prostate tissue, which can lead to difficulty in voiding.

Once the five probes are in place they are activated, allowing liquid nitrogen to flow through the probe. The temperature that is achieved at the probe is $-196°$ C. This causes ice formation on the probe and devitalization of the surrounding prostate tissue. As the five ice balls grow they coalesce into one ovoid ice ball, destroying the prostate tissue in its path. The ice ball also can be extended outside of the prostate gland proper to treat the surrounding tissues of the prostate.

Initial posttreatment biopsies and PSA data have been encouraging.[34,35] The complication rate has varied, and clearly the morbidity associated with the procedure needs to be improved. The complications increased markedly during a time when the federal Food and Drug Administration (FDA) disapproved use of the warming catheter that most cryosurgeons were employing. The catheter has now been placed back in the hands of urologists and once again can be used in patients undergoing cryotherapy. This should decrease the morbidity that occurred when the catheter was unavailable.

There was hope that cryotherapy would allow us to treat patients who had previously undergone radiation treatment but still had persistent disease in the prostate only. Currently, removal of the prostate surgically in these patients presents the patient with a high chance of surgical complications. Also it was hoped that cryotherapy, since it is able to extend outside the prostate, would be a treatment for patients who had T3 disease, since radical prostatectomy and external beam radiation therapy have been unsuccessful in this group of patients.

Currently, cryotherapy should be considered investigational, and the long-term data regarding the effectiveness of the procedure in eradicating prostate cancer are unknown. Further work is needed in refining the technique and developing clearer patient selection criteria. Nevertheless, cryotherapy offers some hope to that group of patients who are not good candidates for conventional treatment for localized prostate cancer.

Androgen Ablation Therapy

Currently, advanced prostate cancer is treated with hormonal manipulation. Testosterone, which is produced mainly in the testicles (95%) and a small portion from the adrenal glands (5%), allows the cancer to proliferate. If the hormone can be eliminated, the cancer has a tendency to go into remission phase for a period of time. This period can vary, but in most patients the remission phase lasts approximately 2 to 3 years.

With time, some of the cells apparently do not respond to hormonal manipulation and continue to progress. Initially, the majority of the patients have a beneficial effect from removal of the testosterone.[4] Occasionally, this effect can be remarkable; even patients with bony metastases have the metastasis apparently disappear. Unfortunately, in most patients the cancer will progress at a later date.

Elimination of testosterone can be achieved through surgical orchiectomy or through chemical means. Leuprolide acetate (Lupron Depot) and metacholine chloride (Zoladex) have been developed to be given in injection form to help "turn off" the production of testosterone. Antiantigen oral medication can also be used to help eliminate the effect of antigens produced by the adrenal gland. Currently, there appears to be some advantage in treating patients both with the injection and the antiantigen over the injection alone. The side effects from the injection or surgical orchiectomy appear to be small. Most patients tolerate the reduction in testosterone very well.

Conclusion

In summary, we have gained a good deal of knowledge to increase our understanding of prostate cancer's natural history and have developed some effective treatments to combat the disease in a localized form. What is needed in the future is a treatment to effectively eradicate the disease once it escapes from the prostate gland. Our ability to detect the cancer earlier has improved markedly since the advent of PSA and transrectal ultrasound needle-guided biopsy. Although no definite proof is available that this will have an impact on our ability to lower the morbidity of prostate cancer, several factors indicate that with time the benefit of early detection should be realized.

Every patient is unique, and each cancer needs to be fully understood regarding its particular characteristics. It is vital that the patient become actively involved with his medical team in deciding the proper and most advantageous treatment for himself.

As a physician I am often amazed at the enduring, tenacious human will to survive. I have seen this in many of my patients who have been diagnosed with prostate cancer. I salute Allen Salowe and the many thousands like him who have demonstrated heroism on a daily basis in facing their disease. This book has explored the extreme importance of the patient's becoming involved in the battle against his own prostate cancer. Allen Salowe is a living testament to how an individual can make a difference in his own treatment.

REFERENCES

1. Parker SL, et al. Cancer 46:4-27, 1996.
2. Steinberg GD, et al. Prostate 17:337-347, 1990.
3. Mebane C, et al. Journal of the National Medical Association 82:782-788, 1990.
4. Huggins C, et al. Cancer Research 1:293, 1941.
5. LePor H, et al. Journal of Urology 128:335, 1982.

6. Halpert B, et al. Cancer 16:737-742, 1963.
7. Giovannucci E, et al. Journal of the American Medical Association 269:878-882, 1993.
8. Giovannucci E, et al. Journal of the American Medical Association 269:873-877, 1993.
9. Bostwick DG, et al. American Cancer Society. Prostate Cancer: What Every Man— and His Family—Needs to Know. New York: Villard Books, 1996.
10. Schmid HP, et al. Cancer 71:2031, 1993.
11. McNeal JE, et al. Human Pathology 23:258, 1992.
12. Chodak B, et al. World Journal of Surgery 13:60, 1989.
13. Thompson IM, et al. World Journal of Surgery 13:65, 1989.
14. Cooner WH. Monographs in Urology 12:3-13, 1991.
15. Crawford ED, et al. Journal of the American Medical Association 267:2227-2228, 1992.
16. Cupp MA, et al. AUA Update 12, Lesson 33, 1993.
17. Catalona WJ, et al. New England Journal of Medicine 324:1156-1161, 1991.
18. Dalkin BL, et al. Journal of Urology 149:413A, 1993.
19. Scardino PT. Urology Clinics of North America 16:635-655, 1989.
20. Benson MC, et al. Journal of Urology 147:817-821, 1992.
21. Clements R, et al. Prostate 4(Suppl):51-56, 1992.
22. Partin AW, et al. Campbell's Urology, 6th ed. Philadelphia: WB Saunders, 1995.
23. Wilson TM, et al. AUA Update 15, Lesson 27, 1996.
24. Gleason DF. Human Pathology 23:273, 1992.
25. Gibbons RP, et al. Journal of Urology 141:564, 1989.
26. LePor H, et al. Journal of Urology 141:82, 1989.
27. Walsh PC, et al. Journal of Urology 128:492, 1982.
28. Igel TC, et al. Journal of Urology 137:1189-1191, 1987.
29. Keetch DW, et al. AUA Update 13:46-51, 1994.
30. Schellhammer P. Monographs in Urology 15:5, 1994.
31. Paulson DF, et al. Journal of Urology 128:502-504, 1982.
32. Johansson JE, et al. Journal of the American Medical Association 267:2191-2196, 1992.
33. Aus G. Scandinavian Journal of Urology and Nephrology 167(Suppl):1-41, 1994.
34. Onik GM, et al. Cancer 72:1291, 1993.
35. Shinohara K, et al. Western Section of the American Urological Association [abstract] 1994.

Summary of Taking Charge Advisories

♦ **The best advice:** Detect prostate disease. Save your life.

1. Ask for a *urologist-administered* digital rectal examination (DRE) and prostate-specific antigen (PSA) blood test.
2. If in doubt, verify the results.
3. Don't delay treatment decisions.
4. Find out what it all means.
5. Broaden your search.
6. Change your doctor if necessary.
7. Get a second opinion.
8. When time is of the essence, demand a quick turnaround.
9. Move your case if that is warranted.
10. Expand your information base.
11. Keep updating the project schedule.
12. Understand that yours is a statistical case of one.
13. Build a positive mind-set.
14. Go for it together.
15. Learn the new tools.
16. Accept.
17. Progress makes perfect.
18. Let nature do some of the work.
19. Occupy the mind in turbulent times.
20. Listen to your body.
21. Adapt to a new lifestyle.

Appendix B

Nine Underlying Principles for Decision Making and Problem Solving

The How and Why of Finding Solutions

Project management is built on reasoning, problem solving, and decision making. Effectively managing the many decisions related to the treatment and healing of prostate cancer, a life-threatening disease, calls for a thorough grasp of the necessary activities. Challenges frequently arise without warning, demanding quick, sure judgment calls—good decisions in a difficult situation. These responses can be summarized as nine underlying principles for carrying out the functions described in this process.

1. Successful people question both *how* and *why* they must spend time and effort to find solutions. This is the basic principle that gives us the key to power. It is an efficient and effective tool for determining how to approach the problem, why you want or need to solve it, and your satisfaction with potential solutions. *Prioritizing expectations helps you deal with new realities.*

2. Every problem exists as a class of one. It is unique because it lies in a framework unlike any other; it is contextually unique. The further we explore the potential result of different treatments, the more this principle takes shape. *It is critically important to put the problem in the right context.*

3. Every problem must be addressed *polyperceptually*, that is, we must deliberately think about a problem and act on a solution after gathering information from various points of view. No single clinical study or professional opinion should suffice in

tackling and solving such a complex problem. *Look at the problem from all angles.*

4. We must be sure that we are working on the *right problem*. Problems have many disguises and aliases. We can only be sure if we explore the meaning of the problem to us and our purposes for exerting time and effort to find solutions. In my case the trade-off between short-term and long-term results was consistently tested. *The patient who loses faith in his future may have no future.*

5. We must try to find what we perceive to be an ideal solution. Breakthroughs in thinking are always strengthened by our working back from some ideal solution. Understanding our priorities helped set the parameters for selecting the most appropriate treatment option. *The way in which a risk is framed can have a major impact on how we react to it.*

6. Every problem is part of a *technically defined mess.* It is always embedded in and interconnected with other problems. It is part of some system. At first it is easy to get caught up in the prevailing wisdom and lose sight of its applicability to the specific case. *It is essential not to lose sight of the facts related to your particular case.*

7. Seeking other points of view is a *cooperative activity.* We must approach it through cooperative competition—seeking believers and doubters. Literature searches, hearing other patients' experiences, and seeking a second opinion set the stage for challenging the original decision. *At the extremes it is very easy, but few cases fit the extremes. In the zone of ambiguity, matters are more complicated because the stakes are so high.*

8. It is possible to suffer *mental indigestion,* or data overload. We must avoid "knowing too much." In its place we must learn how to *structure the information* so it helps us to make an informed decision. *Organize your thoughts. Write them down. Sift and filter often.*

9. Life, like love and liberty, must be won anew; we must regenerate our life-force. The task is not to build up a complicated mix of factors, but rather to *reduce* a large number of initial possibilities to one—the appropriate course of action. *Start from that moment; don't look back.*

Appendix C

Staging and Grading Prostate Cancer

Prostate Cancer Staging

The stage is defined as the mass or bulk of the tumor at the current time. More specifically, how large is the cancer within the prostate, and has it spread to tissues around the prostate or to other parts of the body? The tests employed vary from patient to patient, depending on various factors. The usual initial staging studies include the ultrasound report from the initial biopsy, the pathology report, the DRE, and a bone scan. On occasion, CT scans or MRI evaluations are performed on the pelvic and abdominal areas and a chest x-ray film is evaluated. The stage of the cancer is the most important factor in deciding which treatment to use.

Prostate cancer is now more commonly classified by the tumor-node-metastasis (TNM) system rather than the older Whitmore-Jewett (ABCD) staging system. It is likely that both systems will be encountered in the medical literature, other books, newspaper articles, and medical records.

The TNM System*

T1 *Clinically inapparent tumor, not palpable or visible by imaging*
  T1a Less than 5% of tissue resected (i.e., by TURP)
  T1b More than 5% of tissue resected
  T1c Tumor identified by needle biopsy

*Adapted from Patient Care, April 15, 1995.

T2   *Confined within the prostate*
   T2a   Involving half of a lobe or less
   T2b   More than half a lobe, but not both lobes
   T2c   Both lobes
T3   *Tumor extends through the prostate capsule*
   T3a   Unilateral extracapsular extension
   T3b   Bilateral extracapsular extension
   T3c   Tumor invades seminal vesicles
T4   *Tumor is fixed or invades adjacent structures other than seminal vesicles (N+)*
   T4a   Invades bladder neck and/or external sphincter and/or rectum (M+)
   T4b   Invades levator muscles and/or is fixed in pelvic wall (M+)

The Whitmore-Jewett System*

A1   Well- or moderately well-differentiated tumors involving less than 5% of the tissue, found incidentally when the prostate is resected for presumed benign prostatic hyperplasia (BPH)
A2   Tumors found incidentally, as with A1, but either poorly differentiated or involving more than 5% of the tissue volume
B1   Palpable on rectal examination and confined within the prostate, less than or equal to 2 cm (1 cm = 0.39 inch) and involving only one lobe
B2   Palpable on rectal examination and confined within the prostate, involving one lobe but larger than 2 cm
B3   Palpable on rectal examination, confined within the prostate, but involving both lobes
C1   Extends beyond the boundaries of the prostate, but confined within the pelvis (such as into seminal vesicles or to the pelvic wall), and less than 6 cm
C2   Extends beyond the boundaries of the prostate, but confined within the pelvis (such as into seminal vesicles or to the pelvic wall), and greater than or equal to 6 cm

*Adapted from Patient Care, April 15, 1995, and Harrison's Principles of Internal Medicine, which differ in some details.

> **D0**   Elevated acid phosphatase levels, suggesting metastasis, but without radiographic or physical evidence of this
> **D1**   Metastatic to pelvic lymph nodes
> **D2**   Metastatic to distant sites

Gleason Grading

The grade is determined by the pathologist from the results of the biopsy. The grade provides a gauge of how fast the cancer might be growing or how aggressive it might be. High-grade cancers grow faster and spread earlier than low-grade cancers. Today cancer specialists usually use a Gleason grading system, named after a pathologist from the University of Minnesota. The criteria describe and rate the cancer cells in two ways: (1) how the cancer cells look, and (2) how they are arranged together. Each component is assigned a number from 2 to 5, and the sum of the two numbers is the Gleason score. The urologist may refer to a cancer as a "Gleason 7," or simply a "grade 5," and so on. The higher the number, the worse the cancer. For example, my cancer was determined to be a Gleason 9. Scores range from 2 to 10. They are the sum of the dominant cancer cell patterns, each graded 1 to 5.

> **2-4**   Well-differentiated, cancer cells resemble normal tissue, usually grow gradually
> **5-7**   Moderately differentiated
> **8-10**   Poorly differentiated, do not resemble normal cells, usually grow quickly and spread

To compare systems, physicians say that Gleason 2, 3, and 4 are well differentiated. Grade, while important, may have less bearing on the treatment decisions than the stage. After the grade and stage are known, other factors also come into play before any decision can be made about future treatment. Most important are each individual's health, life expectancy, and current medical conditions, all of which are best determined in consultation with your physician-partner.

Prostate Cancer Resources

American Cancer Society (ACS) (Man to Man Network)
(800) ACS-2345   (800) 227-2345
In Georgia: (404) 320-3333
National Office
1599 Clifton Rd., NE
Atlanta, GA 30329
The prostate cancer Man to Man Network meets monthly in most ACS local chapters, of which there are nearly 3000. Programs available for prostate cancer patients and their families include literature and talks by local specialists who diagnose and treat prostate disease. Call the 800 number or the local chapter of the American Cancer Society in your city or county.

American Foundation for Urologic Disease (A.F.U.D.)
(800) 242-2383
300 W. Pratt St., Suite 401
Baltimore, MD 21201
A.F.U.D. is one of the leading nationwide prostate cancer organizations and concentrates on prostate cancer advocacy, research, and awareness. It has a prostate cancer support network of about 450 affiliated chapters and provides printed material on prevention and treatment of prostate cancer. An 800 call will put you directly in touch with a knowledgeable person to help guide your next steps.

National Cancer Institute
(800) 4-CANCER   (800) 422-6237
Cancer Information Service
National Institutes of Health
Building 31, Room 10A25
Bethesda, MD 20892
The Cancer Information Service, sponsored by the U.S. government as part of the National Institutes of Health, offers one-on-one advice and is available 9:00 AM to 4:30 PM Eastern Time. If you have questions about cancer, they can put you in touch with PDQ, a computer system that provides updated treatment information as well as resources in your area. Up-to-date written reports are available on request.

National Coalition for Cancer Survivorship
(301) 650-8868
1010 Wayne Avenue, Fifth Floor
Silver Springs, MD 20910
The National Coalition for Cancer Survivorship is a network of survivors and related organizations. It provides information regarding local and regional support groups. The coalition works for cancer survivors as an advocate in the workplace, especially concerning discrimination.

Patient Advocates for Advanced Cancer Treatments, Inc. (PAACT)
(616) 453-1477   FAX (616) 453-1846
P.O. Box 141695
Grand Rapids, MI 49154-1695
This group is a clearinghouse and advocacy group for information on prostate cancer treatments. Their representatives are strong proponents of cryosurgery. Your evaluation of the opinions they express should be tempered by the fact that current clinical experience with cryosurgery is limited. This is a good source of clinical reports and patient experiences related to all forms of prostate cancer treatment.

The Prostatitis Foundation
(309) 664-6222
Internet: *www/prostate.org/aboutpf.html*
The Prostatitis Foundation is primarily Internet based. The organization promotes prostatitis research, collects data on the disease, and provides in-

formation and advice to men with the disease. It reports on the proceedings of the annual American Urological Association (AUA) convention. Considerable information can be obtained through their Internet address.

US TOO! International, Inc.
(800) 80-US-TOO   (800) 808-7866
In the Chicago area: (708) 323-1003
FAX (708) 323-1003
930 N. York Rd., Suite 50
Hinsdale, IL 60521-2993
US TOO! International, Inc., is a network of support groups with more than 500 chapters, including some in foreign countries. US TOO! counsels prostate cancer patients to maintain a positive attitude, retain impeccable records of tests, and assume responsibility for their own health by learning everything possible about prostate cancer and its various treatment options and sharing final treatment decisions with their doctor. Chapters conduct support meetings in many states and publish a quarterly newsletter to members. The medical information is monitored by a prestigious medical advisory board.

Board Certification
(800) 776-2378
http://www.ama-assn.org
To determine whether your doctor is board certified, you can call this number. The service is provided by the American Board of Medical Specialties. They receive over 2000 calls per day so you can also call or visit your local library and ask to check the American Medical Association Medical Directory. To determine board certification in urology, call (810) 646-9720; for family practice, call (606) 269-5626. The Web site service provided by the American Medical Association takes you to a free service—AMA Physician Select, which provides a profile of the physician's background and experience.

Prostate Cancer Around the Globe

In recent years prostate cancer has been receiving increasing worldwide attention, in part because it has struck many high-profile political leaders, including the following men:

†François Mitterand, President of France
Moshe Arens, Israeli Defense Minister and former Ambassador to the United States
King Hussein of Jordan
King Norodom Sihanouk of Cambodia
†King Baudoin of Belgium
†Turgol Ozal, President of Turkey
†Felix Houphonet, President of Ivory Coast
†Ayatollah Khomeini, religious and political leader of Iran
Bob Dole, former U.S. senator and 1996 presidential candidate

In Sweden, approximately 25% of all newly diagnosed cancers in men are cancer of the prostate. In the United Kingdom, the incidence of prostate cancer is reportedly on the rise, while the debate over PSA testing quietly goes on. Canadian researchers at the University of Toronto have concluded that testing men with no overt symptoms of prostate cancer is inadvisable, even though the incidence of prostate cancer is on the rise in Canada. A debate also rages in Canada concerning whether the use of the PSA test to screen for the disease is beneficial. A study in Denmark of 73,000 men who had undergone a

†Deceased.

vasectomy between 1977 and 1989 found no evidence that a vasectomy increases the risk of prostate cancer, although they cautioned that in most cases prostate cancer grows very slowly. Research into the effects of a low-fat soy product diet was studied jointly by the University of Helsinki and the National Cancer Research Institute of Tokyo comparing the blood samples and the risk of prostate cancer of Finnish and Japanese men of similar ages. Doctors at St. Bartholomew's Hospital in London reported a new way to diagnose prostate cancer at an early stage, as recently cited in the *Malaysian Doctor*, a professional journal. Researchers at the Institute of Reproduction and Development at Monash University, Australia, are working to understand the exact causes of prostate cancer. Australia recently decided to deemphasize routine PSA testing for men.

As a result of a wide disparity in approaches to prostate cancer diagnosis and treatments, the World Health Organization (WHO) and International Union Against Cancer held the first International Consultation on Prostate Cancer in the summer of 1996. The meetings on prostate cancer covered 18 topics encompassing the field of prostate cancer. Each topic in this ongoing process will be studied by a committee composed of about 10 international experts headed by a chairperson, and each committee will render a written report and recommendations on the particular topic. Among the sponsors of the meeting are the following:

American Cancer Society
American Urological Association
Belgian Urological Association
British Association of Urological Surgeons
Chinese Society of Urology
Danish Urological Society
Dutch Urological Society
European Organization for Research and Treatment of Cancer (EORTC)
European Association of Urology
French Urological Association
German Society of Urology

International Consultation on Urological Diseases
International Continence Society
International Prostate Health Council
International Union Against Cancer
Italian Society of Urology
Japanese Urological Society
Polish Urological Society
SIFUD
Spanish Urological Association
Swiss Society of Urology
Urological Society of Australasia

Helpful Abbreviations

From time to time the patient or his family may come across "medical shorthand"—the abbreviations or acronyms most commonly used in communicating about prostate cancer. Following is a brief guide to some of these terms.

AUA	American Urological Association
BB	Bulletin board (computer bulletin boards)
BPH	Benign prostatic hyperplasia; noncancerous enlargement of the prostate
CaP	*See* PCa
CDUS	Color Doppler ultrasound
cGy	Centigray (a unit of measure in radiology)
CHB	Complete or combined hormonal blockade
CHT	Complete or combined hormonal therapy
Cryo	Cryoblation of the prostate (surgical removal of the prostate by a freezing process)
DRE	Digital rectal examination
MRI	Magnetic resonance imaging
PAP	Prostatic acid phosphatase
PBR	Proton beam radiation
PCa	Prostate cancer (also abbreviated CaP)
PSA	Prostate-specific antigen (PCa screening blood test)
RP	Radical prostatectomy (surgical removal of the prostate)
RT	Radiation therapy (bombardment of cancer cells with x-rays)
TRUS	Transrectal ultrasound
TURP	Transurethral resection of the prostate
URL	Uniform resource locator (used in Internet searches)
WW	Watchful waiting
WWW	WorldWide Web (Internet resources)

Toward a National Prostate Cancer Coalition

M. Brooke Moran

Since 1992, the number of American men diagnosed with prostate cancer per year has risen from approximately 132,000 to 317,000, according to the American Cancer Society. This staggering increase can be attributed to the following factors:

- Increased public awareness of men's health issues, including prostate diseases
- Improved testing methods for prostate cancer, especially through the use of the DRE combined with the PSA blood test
- National awareness campaigns, such as Prostate Cancer Awareness Week
- Prominent individuals who have come forward and identified themselves as prostate cancer survivors (Bob Dole, Norman Schwarzkopf, Arnold Palmer, etc.)
- The graying of the baby boomers

Unfortunately, the media continue to focus on prostate cancer being a "man's disease," forgetting to focus on the family that stands with these men and the future generations that will be affected by the diagnosis of prostate cancer in families. *The message that prostate cancer is a disease that profoundly affects the American family is not being heard.*

Federal research allocations for prostate cancer have not risen proportionately with the increase in the number of men diagnosed with the disease. In fact, federal research allocations have been quite small when compared with those for diseases of similar incidence and mortality, such as AIDS and breast cancer (Figure 7). In 1996, federal research allocations exceeded $1.6 billion for AIDS research, $550 million for breast cancer research, and approximately $80 million for prostate cancer research.

Why is there such a discrepancy in federal research allocations? Why have federal research allocations been so low, although the mortality rate is almost equal and the incidence is so much higher? The answer is simple: "The squeaky wheel gets the oil." After making numerous visits to legislators on Capitol Hill, this was the message that was heard. The AIDS and breast cancer patient communities were ex-

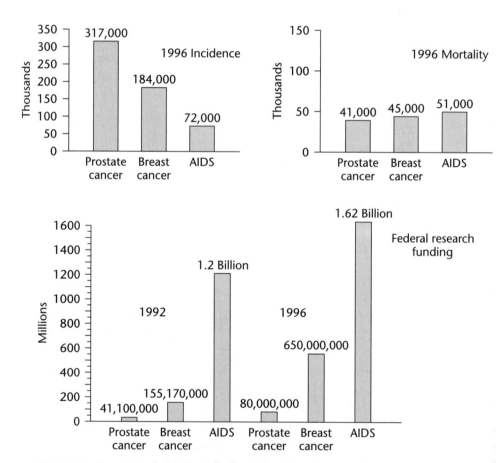

Figure 7 Comparison of federal research allocations for prostate cancer, breast cancer, and AIDS.

tremely effective in coming together and bringing their messages to Congress and the American public.

AIDS and breast cancer are perceived as diseases of "epidemic" proportions and threats to the health and welfare of our country. The AIDS communities were the first activists to band together and advocate change in public attitudes and policies toward that disease. The federal government responded to their battle cry, and now billions of federal dollars are earmarked for AIDS research, education, and support.

Betty Ford is credited with bringing breast cancer out of the closet in 1981, when she publicly acknowledged and openly discussed her own breast cancer and urged women everywhere to learn breast self-examination and to seek regular breast examinations from health care professionals. Before that time, we maintained an almost Victorian attitude, avoiding the mention of certain body parts in public. For instance, do you remember how your grandparents referred to the "white and dark meat" of Sunday's chicken dinner or the Thanksgiving turkey. This was the Victorian way of avoiding the words "breast" and "thigh." Betty Ford's publicized battle with breast cancer started a parade of women coming forward and stating that they too were breast cancer survivors. This parade has never ended.

In times of crisis, women band together in small groups or "circles" to support each other and to share their experiences. Many breast cancer survivors began meeting in small groups of twos, threes, and fours. These groups began to grow and formalize into support or "self-help" groups. (In the technical argot self-help groups are run and facilitated by the members themselves, whereas support groups are facilitated by a professional, such as a social worker.) As the women came together, they made a startling discovery. These women, who are now in their late forties and fifties, many of whom had been activists in the 1960s, found that their daughters were now being diagnosed with breast cancer. To their dismay, these younger women were being presented with the same treatment options that had been available to their mothers 5, 10, and 15 years before. Nothing new seemed to have taken place for breast cancer research or treatment. This promoted anger.

A very fine line separates anger from passion. The passion of the breast cancer survivors quickly shifted to anger as they perceived the lack of progress in breast cancer research for over a generation. In 1991, more than 140,000 petitions were brought to the White House demanding that breast cancer receive the highest American health care priority. The petitions were carried into the White House by security guards. Unfortunately, the breast cancer activists were not invited inside. To this day, they have no idea what happened to those original petitions.

That experience inflamed them to more anger and passion to bring breast cancer to the forefront of public attention. The activists realized that a collective organization, a coalition, was needed to bring about a change in the public attitude toward breast cancer. Thus in 1991 the National Breast Cancer Coalition (NBCC) was formed. The threefold mission of the NBCC is to cure breast cancer "through increased research, improved access to detection and treatments, and to be an influence in the federal decision making processes regarding the disease."

An initial organized petition drive, "Do the Write Thing," generated over 600,000 signatures in 6 weeks. A second petition drive in 1992, entitled "1 in 8," meaning that one in every eight women will be diagnosed with breast cancer, generated more than 2.6 million signatures in 6 months. The NBCC leadership personally took the petitions into the White House this time. No more peering through the palings at those in a position of power.

The NBCC became an effective and highly creditable lobbying agent on Capitol Hill. Through its efforts, federal research dollars earmarked for breast cancer rose from $82 million in 1981 to more than $550 million in 1996. More than 350 organizations plus thousands of individuals are members of the NBCC. Its grassroots advocacy network of volunteers has the capacity to shut down a legislator's communications system in 30 minutes with calls, faxes, and e-mails in response to a particular stand on breast cancer–related legislation.

Relating the Breast Cancer Experience to Prostate Cancer Efforts

How does this brief description of the formation of the NBCC relate to prostate cancer? If the time is moved forward 10 years, the comparisons are striking.

In 1991, "prostate" was not a household word. If asked in a "man on the street" interview, few people knew what a "prostate" was, who had one, where they could find one, or what it did. All this is changing.

In December 1991, Senator Bob Dole acknowledged that he had been diagnosed with prostate cancer and had recently had a radical prostatectomy. His message was this:

Men, you owe it to yourselves and your families to be checked for prostate cancer with a PSA and a DRE. Through these tests, I was diagnosed with prostate cancer in its early, treatable stages. After considering all the treatment options, my physician and I made an educated treatment decision. I've had my treatment, now I'm moving ahead with my life. Men, get checked for prostate cancer!

Senator Dole's drive and stamina to withstand the rigors of a presidential campaign give testimony to his good health since his surgery. Since Senator Dole's revelation, General Norman Schwarzkopf, Sidney Poitier, Michael Milken, Robert Goulet, and sports figures Len Dawson, Bob Watson, Arnold Palmer, and Marv Levy have joined the list of public figures who have acknowledged their diagnosis of prostate cancer.

Senator Dole's message hit home with men and their wives all over the country. More and more men were making appointments to have their prostates checked through the use of PSAs and DREs. Wives and partners were pushing men into their physicians' offices. Although the number of men being diagnosed was increasing, the number of men being diagnosed with late-stage disease was increasing at a much lower rate. Men were being diagnosed and treated for prostate cancer before symptoms had begun to manifest themselves. Prostate cancer treatments, however, were prone to leave side effects on their patients—side effects that a man could have for the rest of his life and that could seriously affect his quality and outlook on life.

The prostate cancer survivors, like their breast cancer counterparts, began forming support and self-help groups to learn more about their collective disease and to support each other and their families through the crises and for the long haul.

Many of the original groups, such as Man to Man and US TOO!, were formed by urologists and patients working together. Man to Man has since become part of the American Cancer Society and is being developed by their regional divisions across the country. From 1991 to 1996, the numbers of local prostate cancer support groups around the country grew from a handful to hundreds.

Recognizing the success of the NBCC in bringing breast cancer to the public's attention, and understanding that federal funding for prostate cancer must be stepped up dramatically, the American Foundation for Urologic Disease (A.F.U.D.) called a task force of representatives of all prostate cancer organizations, leading prostate cancer patients and advocates, to form a national prostate cancer coalition. Jon Huntsman, president of Huntsman Cancer Institute of Salt Lake City and a prostate cancer survivor who is totally dedicated to increasing cancer research, was the honorary chairman.

Jane Reese-Coulburne, vice president of the NBCC, gave a keynote speech that brought the attendees to their feet and made the word "inclusive" a part of the formation document and premise of the now-formed National Prostate Cancer Coalition (NPCC). The mission of the NPCC, "the elimination of prostate cancer as a disease of serious concern for men and their families," brings home the fact that we may never find a total "cure" for prostate cancer. We must, however, bring the message to the American public that prostate cancer is a disease that has a major and often devastating impact on the lives of *American families*. Then, we will create the passion necessary to bring public attention to prostate cancer to enable scientists to discover better means of detection, prevention, and the eventual cure of the disease.

The formation of the NPCC included and encouraged both men and women. The men have proved to be planners, whereas the women have brought activism and passion to the organization. All this is necessary if we are to climb mountains.

For information on participation and membership in the National Prostate Cancer Coalition, please write:
National Prostate Cancer Coalition
1300 19th Street, NW
Suite 400
Washington, DC 20036

♦
_____

Glossary

Finding the right words to describe your pain, discomfort, or physical performance will go a long way in helping your doctor find the right diagnosis and treatment. With just a little bit of extra effort you can become familiar with the language of prostate cancer screening, treatment, and healing. The use of this specialized language helps enhance understanding between the patient and physician. Armed with the proper terminology, you will be increasingly comfortable talking directly with your physician-partner, and he or she will be able to explain clinical findings in more specific detail when you grasp the terms.

First, in describing your symptoms, begin with the basics and describe the location, intensity, frequency, and what makes matters better or worse. Next, convey the quality of your pain or discomfort (feeling). Words such as *stinging, penetrating, dull, throbbing, aching, nagging,* or *gnawing* may give your doctor a clearer understanding of your physical discomfort.

Once the pain has passed, it is difficult to reconstruct your precise sensation in words. Therefore keep a urologic or pain diary so that you can write down a detailed description of your pain or discomfort while you still have it.

Although the language of prostate cancer may arise anywhere along the screening-treatment-healing continuum, we repeatedly came across certain key words in readings and conversation. Such terms are preceded by a bullet (•) for emphasis.

A

- **abdomen** The lower part of the trunk of the body, which contains such vital organs as the intestines, liver, stomach, and spleen.

  abdominal aortic aneurysm (AAA) Abnormal swelling and weakening of the large arterial trunk that carries blood from the heart to the rest of the body.

  acid phosphatase A substance made in the prostate gland.

- **acute** Having a sudden onset and (usually) a short, severe course.

- **adenocarcinoma** Cancer derived from abnormal gland cells from the lining of an organ. Most prostate cancers are of the adenocarcinoma type.

- **adjunctive therapy** The addition of radiation, hormone therapy, or chemotherapy after surgery. Hormone therapy is also used before surgery to shrink the enlarged prostate gland.

- **adrenal (uh-DREE-nal) glands** Secretory organs located above each kidney that produce several kinds of hormones, including the sex hormones that can feed prostate cancer. Adjunctive hormone therapy is used to block production of testosterone.

- **age adjusted** Adaptation of laboratory results so that they appropriately relate to a patient's age, an important consideration when evaluating treatment alternatives relative to the patient's *normal* life expectancy.

  alkaline phosphatase Enzyme produced in the liver and bones that is measured to help determine whether prostate cancer has spread to the bones.

  anaphylactic reaction Sudden, life-threatening reaction to a substance or medication.

- **androgen (AN-dro-jen)** A hormonal substance necessary for the development and functioning of the male sex organs and male sexual characteristics such as deep voice and facial hair.

- **androgen blockade** A barrier to male hormone production. Before the cryoablation of the prostate procedure was developed, androgen blockade was used to debulk the prostate.

- **anesthesia** Induction of a state in which pain cannot be felt, by use of a medication or anesthetic agent, such as during a surgical procedure.

- **anterior** The front of an organ or structure.

  antibiotic A medication used to inhibit the growth of or kill microorganisms that can cause an infection.

- **antiandrogen** Medication that reduces or eliminates the presence or activity of androgens in the body.

- **anti-inflammatory** Medication that reduces pain, swelling, redness, and irritation from injury, surgery, or infection.

  anus (A-nus) The external terminus of the rectum.

- **apex** The tip of the prostate gland located farthest from the bladder.

- **artificial urinary sphincter (SFINK-ter)** A surgically implanted prosthetic device activated by the patient to compress the urethra and reduce urinary leakage (one of several alternatives to help control permanent incontinence).

  aspiration Removal of fluid or tissue by using suction, usually through a fine needle.

- **autologous transfusion** Using a person's own blood for blood transfusion, if necessary, during surgery.

B

- **bacteria** One-celled microorganisms that can cause infection under certain conditions.

  balloon dilation An abandoned technique, formerly used to stretch open the prostate to improve urine flow.

  base Wide part of the prostate adjacent to the bladder.

- **benign (be-NINE)** A growth that is not cancerous. Such tissue generally does not spread to other organs or come back when removed.

  beta-carotene A nutrient found in dark-yellow and dark-green leafy vegetables; important for normal health.

- **biopsy** Surgical removal of small tissue samples for microscopic examination to determine whether cancer is present; the most essential investigative step when the PSA level is elevated or a DRE reveals suspicious characteristics.

- **bladder** Muscular, hollow organ in which urine is stored before it is discharged from the body. The bladder is important to the healing process after prostate surgery.

- **bladder neck** Circular muscle fibers that come together like a funnel where the bladder opens into the prostate.

- **bladder spasms** Painful clenching of the bladder muscles in response to irritation or injury.

- **blood clot** Thickening of blood to form a semisolid mass inside a blood vessel. A postoperative blood clot may form that the body most often expels.

- **blood count** Measurement of the number of blood cells in given volume of blood. Red cells (erythrocytes) carry oxygen to the tissues; white cells (leukocytes) produce macrophages and antibody-producing lymphoctyes to fight infection.

  bone marrow The spongy material inside the bones that produces red blood cells.

- **bone scan** A type of nuclear medicine scan that allows a sensitive look at the entire skeleton for any changes that might suggest metastatic spread of prostate cancer. This is often the next diagnostic measure after a biopsy finding of cancer.

• **bowel preparation** Cleansing of the intestines before abdominal surgery by use of a cathartic agent; also called bowel prep.

• **benign prostatic hyperplasia (BPH)** Noncancerous enlargement of the prostate that may cause difficulty in urination; the most common aging-related experience for all men.

• **brachytherapy (BRAKE-ee-THER-a-pee)** Radiation therapy in which radioactive pellets are inserted into the prostate; a fairly recent treatment alternative with promising 5-year survival history.

C

• **cancer** Abnormal and uncontrolled growth of cells in the body; also called a malignant tumor, neoplasm, or carcinoma. Cancer can spread to other parts of the body and ultimately injure and kill.

• **capsule** Fibrous outer lining of the prostate.

carcinoma Cancer.

castration Surgical removal of the testicles; *see also* orchiectomy.

• **catheter** A hollow tube used to drain fluids from or inject fluids into body cavities.

cell-saver Machine used to recycle blood lost during surgery and give it back to the patient during the procedure.

cell Smallest unit of the body. Cells make up tissues.

chemoprevention Use of a substance to prevent the development and growth of cancer.

chemotherapy (kee-mo-THER-a-pee) Cancer treatment utilizing various powerful drugs to attack and destroy certain kinds of cancer.

• **chronic** Persisting over a long period of time.

• **clinical trials** Use of a new medication or treatment under strict controls to determine whether the new therapy is safe and effective. At this writing, numerous clinical trials for prostate cancer are underway throughout the world.

colostomy Surgical opening of the large intestine to the skin, with drainage of the bowel contents into a bag.

• **complication** A secondary condition or disease arising during the course of a primary condition; for example, scarring of the bladder neck after prostate surgery causes narrowing of the passage.

• **cryotherapy or cryosurgery** Freezing of the prostate, which results in surgical destruction of the prostate (still an investigational procedure that holds promise); also called cryoablation.

- **CT (or CAT) scan** Computed axial tomography; a computerized x-ray scan of the body that shows the internal organs in a cross-sectional view to visualize abnormalities.

cystitis An inflammatory condition of the bladder that is often caused by infection.

- **cystoscope** Fiberoptic instrument used to look inside the bladder and urethra.

D

debridement (de-BREED-ment or day-BREED-maw) Removal of contaminated or devitalized tissue from adjacent tissue until surrounding healthy tissue is exposed.

- **debulk** To reduce the volume of the prostate by surgery, hormone therapy, or chemotherapy (before the development of cryosurgery, hormone therapy was used to debulk the prostate gland; the 20% size reduction improved the target area for placement of probes).

deep venous thrombosis Formation of a clot in the large, deep veins, usually of the pelvis or legs.

deferred therapy Delaying treatment until cancer becomes a definite threat to the patient; also called watchful waiting. This approach should *only* be taken after consultation with the doctor.

- **diagnosis** Determination of the cause or existence of a medical problem or disease.

diet regular eating and drinking habits; specifically, what a person eats.

- **digital rectal examination (DRE)** An examination of the prostate gland through the rectum by the physician's lubricated, gloved finger. It is a recommended annual event for every man over age 50 and beginning annually for men over 40 with a family history of prostate cancer. It takes only a few seconds, is painless, and may save a man's life.

dihydrotestosterone (DHT) Active breakdown product of testosterone; more powerful than testosterone.

directed donations Blood donated by friends or family for a patient with the intention that it can be used for transfusion if necessary.

dissection Surgical cutting of tissue.

double-blind Research study in which neither doctor nor patient knows what medication or treatment is being used.

- **doubling time** Length of time for a set volume of cancer to double in size, an important measure of periodic changes in PSA level (a good reason for every man to know his annual PSA number and calculate the rate of change from test to test).

downsize To shrink or reduce the size of the cancerous tumor.

• **downstage** To reduce the initial stage of a cancer to a lower (and presumably better) stage; for example, from stage B to stage A.

E

epidural anesthesia Anesthesia in which a powerful narcotic drips directly into the fluid that surrounds the spinal cord. This results in blockage of pain while allowing normal sensation and muscle function; commonly used in childbirth.

• **ejaculation** Release of semen from the penis during sexual climax.

• **erectile dysfunction** Any abnormality in achieving or maintaining a penile erection (sometimes used synonymously with impotence).

estrogen (ES-tro-jin) Female hormone.

estrogen therapy Use of estrogen pills to block the male hormones as a treatment for advanced prostate cancer.

• **Eulexin** Trade name for flutamide; *see also* flutamide.

experimental Untested or unproved treatment or approach (sometimes used synonymously with investigational, although technically they do not mean the same thing).

external vacuum device A plastic tube used with a suction appliance to produce an erection; used as a treatment for impotence.

F

family physician Primary care doctor who treats all members of the family; formerly called a general practitioner.

fiberoptics New technology that allows looking at internal structures through fine fibers inside of an instrument.

• **flutamide (FLU-ta-mide)** A medication in tablet form taken three times a day to provide total androgen blockage, that is, blocking any remaining adrenal androgens from the cells (10 days' usage, together with 3 months of shots, may constitute a presurgical regimen).

• **Foley catheter** Latex or silicone tube that drains urine from the bladder to an outside collection bag; commonly used temporarily after prostate surgery to empty the bladder and allow postsurgical healing to begin.

• **frequency** The need to urinate often. This is an early symptom of a possible prostate problem that men frequently overlook and consider unimportant. It needs to be checked out early.

• **frozen section** Preliminary rapid analysis of tissue by a pathologist who freezes the sample so that a thin slice can be shaved off to use in microscopic examination; *see also* permanent section.

G

gatekeeper Primary care physician, usually associated with an HMO, who controls referrals of patients to specialists for tests and evaluations.

general anesthesia A state of consciousness induced before surgery with anesthetic agents, producing a generalized insensibility to pain and a degree of muscle relaxation.

• **genetics** Branch of science that studies inherited characteristics (there is a strong causal link between the incidence of prostate cancer and male family members).

• **genitourinary tract** The urinary system (kidney, ureters, bladder, and urethra) and the genital system (testicles, vas deferens, prostate, and penis).

• **gland** Structure or organ that produces a substance to be used in another part of the body (the prostate is a gland).

goserelin acetate Luteinizing hormone–releasing hormone (LH-RH) medication in pellet form. It is inserted just under the skin every 28 days to lower the testosterone level for the treatment of advanced prostate cancer.

• **grade** In cancer, the descriptive designation of the degree of malignancy based on the microscopic appearance of the cells.

groin Region of the body at which the legs attach to the torso on the lower abdomen.

gynecomastia Enlargement of the male breast, often accompanied by tenderness; can occur on one side or both.

H

health maintenance organization (HMO) A network system of contracted health care providers who offer medical care to an enrolled group of patients.

hematospermia Blood in the semen.

hematuria Blood in the urine.

heparin A widely used anticoagulant (that is, blood-thinning, anticlotting) medication.

heparin lock A device placed into an intravenous line that is being used for heparin administration. The lock is periodically flushed to ensure patency (openness) of the line.

• **heredity** Transmission of characteristics from parents to children through genetic material (an extremely important consideration among male family members regarding prostate cancer incidence).

hernia Bulging of abdominal contents through a weakness in the abdominal wall, often in the groin.

- **hesitancy** Inability to start the urinary stream immediately.
- **high grade** Very advanced cancer cells.
- **high risk** Having characteristics that make one more likely to have a complication or side effect.
- **hormones** Substances carried in the body that have a regulatory function on certain organs; responsible for secondary sex characteristics.
- **hot flashes** Sudden feelings of warmth, often accompanied by sweating and flushing of the skin, following hormone treatment.

hyperthermia Heating of the prostate to destroy prostate tissue; a fairly recently developed method to relieve the symptoms of benign prostatic hyperplasia.

I

ICU Intensive care unit; section of the hospital in which critically ill patients or those requiring intensive observation and care are placed.

imaging The production of clarity, contrast, and detail to visualize a deep structure of the body through the use of x-rays, magnetic fields, or other means.

immune system Complex system of organs, tissues, blood cells, and substances to resist infection, cancers, and foreign proteins.

- **impotence (IM-po-tens)** Inability to achieve and maintain an erection (one of the potential aftereffects of prostate cancer treatment, whether by prostatectomy, radiation, or cryosurgery).

incision Cutting of the skin at the beginning of a surgical operation.

- **incontinence (in-KON-ti-nens)** Leaking of a substance, as in urinary incontinence (a potential side effect of prostate cancer treatment, regardless of treatment type).

infection A condition resulting from the presence of bacteria or other microorganisms.

- **inflammation** Swelling, pain, redness, and irritation as a result of injury or infection.
- **informed consent** Permission, almost always in writing, given for a treatment by a person who is aware of the possible benefits as well as the potential risks and complications.

inpatient A person admitted to a hospital overnight.

internist A primary care physician who specializes in disease prevention and the nonsurgical management of disease.

- **interstitial (in-ter-STISH-el)** Within an organ; for example, interstitial radiation, in which radioactive seeds are inserted into the prostate.

intravenous Into the veins.

- **invasive** Not just the surface; moving beyond the organ of origin and into other tissues.

investigator Doctor or scientist involved in research and experimental studies of a treatment or medication.

intravenous pyelogram (IVP) X-ray evaluation of the urinary system after a contrast agent is injected that enables the doctor to see images of the kidneys, ureters, and bladder.

K

• **Kegel (KAY-gel) exercises** Pelvic exercises used to treat urinary incontinence. Alternating relaxation and contraction helps to strengthen the muscles used to control urination (an almost certain need as one gets older, especially after prostate treatment); also used following childbirth to restore perineal muscle tone.

kidneys Two large bean-shaped structures that remove waste from the blood.

L

laser Very concentrated beam of high-energy light used in surgery; originally an acronym for *l*ight *a*mplification by *s*timulated *e*mission of *r*adiation.

• **leuprolide acetate** A synthetic substance resembling luteinizing hormone–releasing hormone (LH-RH) that causes the brain to stop stimulating testosterone production.

lymph (limf) A nearly clear fluid collected from the tissues and returned to the blood via the lymphatic system.

• **lymph nodes** Small bean-shaped structures scattered along the vessels of the lymphatic system. The nodes filter bacteria and cancer cells that may travel through the system.

lymphatic (lim-FAT-ik) system Vessels that carry lymph, together with lymph nodes and several organs that produce and store infection-fighting cells.

M

• **magnetic resonance imaging (MRI)** An imaging system employing a tube-shaped chamber into which a person is placed for visualizing internal body structures (the device does *not* use x-rays).

• **malignancy** Uncontrolled growth of cells that can invade and destroy body organs and cause death.

• **malignant (muh-LIG-nant)** Cancerous, with the potential for uncontrolled growth and destruction.

• **metastatic (meh-tu-STAT-ik) cancer** Cancer that has spread to other organs or tissues through the lymphatic or blood system (doctors say the cancer has metastasized).

- **microscopic** Small enough that a microscope is needed to see.
- **moderately differentiated** Intermediate grade of cancer as determined by pathologic analysis of tissue.

N

- **negative** A test result indicating that a particularly sought abnormality is not present.
  neoadjuvant A cancer treatment that precedes a second modality of therapy, such as radiation, hormone therapy, or chemotherapy before surgery; also called adjunctive therapy.
- **neoplastic** malignant, cancerous.
  nephrostomy tube Small tube placed into the kidney through the skin that allows drainage of urine from the kidney.

O

  obturator nerve A large nerve that courses through the pelvis and transmits impulses controlling some leg movements.
- **oncologist (ong-KOHL-o-jist)** A physician who specializes in the evaluation and treatment of cancer.
- **orchiectomy (or-kee-EK-tuh-mee)** Surgical removal of the testicles.
  organs Tissues that work together for a specific function, such as bladder, heart, or kidneys.
- **outpatient** Patient who undergoes surgery or other treatment but does not stay overnight in the hospital.

P

- **pathologist (pah-THOL-o-jist)** Specialty-trained physician who examines tissues under a microscope to determine what they are and whether disease is present (pathologists also oversee laboratory tests, such as PSA blood tests).
  pelvis Region of the body that forms a bony girdle joining the lower limbs of the body.
- **penile (pee-nile)** Relating to the penis.
- **penile prosthesis (pros-THEE-sis)** Surgically implanted device to provide erections for men who have become impotent.
- **perineum (pair-ih-NE-um)** Area just behind the scrotum, in front of the anus (during cryosurgery probes are inserted into the perineum; some surgeons perform prostatectomies through the perineum).
  permanent section Formal preparation of tissue by a pathologist for microscopic analysis; *see also* frozen section.
  placebo Fake medication or treatment with no interactions with the body (often used in research studies to test the efficacy of a new medication).

ploidy status The genetic status of cancer cells; similar to grade.

pneumatic sequential stockings Inflatable stockings that squeeze the legs intermittently to help reduce the risks of serious blood clots.

• **poorly differentiated** High-grade, aggressive cancer, as determined by pathologic analysis of tissue.

• **positive biopsy** The detection of cancer by a biopsy procedure.

• **positive margin** Conditions in which cancer cells are found at the cut edge of tissue removed during surgery (a positive margin indicates that residual cancer may be remaining in the body).

posterior Behind or toward the back.

• **prognosis** Act of foretelling the course of a disease (the long-term outlook or prospect for survival and recovery).

• **progression** Continued growth of the cancer or the disease.

• **prostate** A gland of the male reproductive system that surrounds the urethra located at the base of the bladder that produces some of the sperm-carrying fluid of the semen.

• **prostatectomy (prah-stah-TEK-toe-mee)** Surgical removal of part or all of the prostate gland; used to mean radical (total) removal of the prostate.

• **prostate-specific antigen (anti-jen) (PSA)** Protein secreted by prostate cells (a PSA test helps detect and follow prostate cancer and its importance as a life-saving measure cannot be overstated).

prostatic acid phosphatase (PAP) A chemical once used to try to determine when prostate cancer had spread outside of the gland.

prostatic intraductal neoplasia (PIN) An abnormal area seen in biopsied tissue that is not cancerous but may become cancerous; may indicate that cancer is present in neighboring tissue.

• **prostatitis** Inflammation of the prostate.

prostatodynia Pain in or near the prostate.

prosthesis Artificial device used to replace the lost normal function of a structure or an organ.

• **protocol** An explicit, detailed plan of an experiment or research study to evaluate a specific treatment or medication.

pulmonary embolism Blood clot that travels along the large veins of the body up to the lungs (these can be instantly fatal if large enough).

R

• **radiation (ray-de-AY-shun) therapy** Treatment using x-rays to destroy cancerous tissues; also called radiotherapy.

• **radical prostatectomy** Removal of the prostate gland and surrounding tissues and structures to eliminate cancer; called the "gold standard" of treatment for grade A and B cancers.

• **radioactive seeds** Small pellets of various substances that are treated to become radioactive; when inserted into the body, intended to kill adjacent cancer cells (a recent treatment alternative with promising 5-year results).

• **radiologist** Physician who specializes in performing and interpreting various types of x-ray studies.

randomized Assignment of subjects in an experiment to treatment groups by a random pattern.

recovery room Hospital unit to which patients are transferred after surgery to recover before being sent to their rooms or homes, depending on the type of operation.

rectum Last few inches of the colon leading to the anus.

recurrence Return of disease.

regional recurrence Return of cancer in the same general area where it was first located; *see also* local occurrence.

remission Disappearance of the signs and symptoms of a disease; can be temporary or permanent.

resectoscope A tube-shaped instrument used by the urologist to cut out prostate tissue through the urethra, under direct vision.

resistance Ability to fight off a challenge (some microorganisms have developed a resistance to certain antibiotics; the body has a resistance to infection).

• **retention** Inability to urinate.

• **retropubic (reh-tro-PYOO-bik)** Behind the pubic bone.

risk Chance or probability of something happening.

S

sampling error (SE) In testing, when a problem exists but is not detected by the test.

• **scrotum (SKRO-tum)** Sac that holds the testicles.

selenium An element found in small amounts in food; may have anticancer effects.

semen (SEE-men) Fluid containing sperm that comes out of the penis during ejaculation.

• **seminal vesicles (SEM-en-ul VES-uh-kels)** Glands at the base of the bladder that add nutrients to the semen.

• **sepsis** Systemic infection characterized by high fever and shaking chills.

• **side effect** A secondary, usually adverse, reaction to a medication or treatment.

• **signs** Physical changes that can be observed by the patient or physicians; occur as a result of a disease or disorder. *Compare* symptoms.

simulation Technique using x-rays to plan radiation treatment for prostate cancer.

soy products Products made from the soy bean (a legume).

• **spasm** Rhythmic squeezing that can be painful, such as a bladder spasm.

spermine Substance found in the prostate that slows the growth of prostate cancer.

• **sphincter (SFINK-ter) muscle of urinary bladder** A circular muscle at the bottom of the bladder that under normal conditions prevents urine leakage.

• **spinal anesthesia** Loss of sensation below the level of injection of medication on the spinal cord.

• **stage** Description of the size or quantity of a cancer and the extent of its spread from its original site (stage A and B lesions remain contained within the gland and are usually small; stage C cancer has broken through the prostate wall and is quite large; a stage D tumor has escaped and spread to tissue elsewhere in the body).

stent Tube that allows drainage from one place to another.

• **stricture** A decrease in the caliber of a passage or opening in the body, as when scarring narrows the urethra.

• **suprapubic (SOOP-ra-PYU-bik)** Above the pubic bone, as in a suprapubic incision or catheter.

• **symptoms** Conditions that accompany or result from a disease or disorder (the patient *feels* or experiences a symptom). *Compare* signs.

• **systemic** Throughout the body.

T

• **testicles (TES-ti-kuls)** Two glands located in the scrotum; they produce sperm, testosterone and other sex hormones.

testicular (tes-TIK-U-lar) Relating to the testicles.

• **testosterone (tes-TOS-ter-own)** Primary male sex hormone.

• **therapy** Treatment of a disorder.

thrombosis Formation of a vein-obstructing clot (thrombus).

• **tissue** An aggregate of cells that form structures within the body, such as muscle, cartilage, or hair.

• **total androgen blockade** Total blockage of all male hormones through surgery and/or medications.

transferrin Chemical substance in the body that has been shown to stimulate prostate cancer growth.

• **transperineal** Through the perineum, just under the scrotum and above the anus; describes the entry point for the freezing probes used in cryosurgery.

transrectal Through the rectum.

• **transrectal ultrasound (TRUS)** Ultrasonographic technique used to visualize the prostate gland and to guide biopsy of prostatic tissue.

• **transurethral (trans-yu-REETH-rul) resection of the prostate (TURP)** Surgical technique in which the patient is placed under general anesthesia, then through a fiberoptic instrument with a camera the physician is able to view the prostatic region to determine whether prostate tissue is impeding urine flow from the bladder. A portion of the prostate tissue is removed with the instrument, leaving only the shell of the prostate behind. Some compare this to the coring of an apple.

• **tumor** abnormal tissue growth that can be benign (noncancerous) or malignant (cancerous).

tumor markers Chemical substances in the blood that can be used to detect and follow the treatment of certain cancer.

• **tumor volume** Amount of cancer present in an organ.

U

undergrading Term indicating that the grade of cancer is worse than that found in biopsied tissue (an A might be reclassified as a B or C after removal and laboratory analysis).

ultrasound A technique of visualizing internal organs by measuring reflected sound waves.

unit Term referring to a pint of blood.

ureters (YUR-e-ters) Two thin muscular tubes that carry urine from the kidneys to the bladder.

• **urethra (yu-REETH-rah)** In men, the thin muscular tube that carries urine from the bladder and semen from the prostate and other sex glands out through the tip of the penis.

• **urgency** The compelling urge to urinate.

• **urinalysis** Examination of the urine; part of routine examinations to check for infection or other foreign bacteria.

• **urinary incontinence** A condition in which a person is unable to hold urine and prevent its leakage.

• **urinary retention** Inability to urinate, with the bladder filling with urine.

urine A liquid produced by the kidneys containing the waste and water from the blood.

urine culture A procedure in which bacteria from infected urine are grown and tested in the laboratory

• **urologist (yur-AHL-o-jist)** A doctor who specializes in diseases of the genitourinary tract in men and women (the specialist who deals with prostate cancer).

urostomy A surgical opening that allows urine to drain directly to the skin of the lower abdomen, and then into a collection bag (performed when the bladder is removed and is *not* part of the prostate treatment regimen).

V

• **vas deferens** Tiny tube that conveys sperm from the testicles to the prostate gland.

W

• **well differentiated** Low-grade cancer, as determined by pathologic analysis of tissue.

Z

Zoladex Trade name for goserelin acetate; *see also* goserelin acetate.

♦

Bibliography

There are several good technical guides to prostate cancer as well as books written by survivors who have related their personal experiences with physicians and different treatments. Some are detailed references, whereas others offer a patient's point of view or a personal rather than a clinical view of the disease. I advise you to consider carefully whether a book you are selecting focuses primarily on the man's retaining his potency postoperatively rather than helping him to concentrate on which treatment best increases his chance of *beating* this disease.

A book should become a valuable resource, and we are fortunate to have so many from which to choose. The patient and family need an effective discussion to better understand the different issues surrounding the dilemmas and treatment of prostate cancer. Books of 300 pages or more may prove an overwhelming task for a new patient and family faced with the fast-moving and changing events confronting them in the critical first days and weeks after diagnosis, but may serve them well as an ongoing reference tool.

Consider one or more books written for patients by a survivor with physician input (noted below with an *S*). Look for sharp, clear language that describes the many aspects of dealing with prostate cancer. Scan the book to see whether it conveys basic medical information about the disease and treatment in a straightforward, nontechnical manner and whether it can be read in an evening.

Altman, Roberta. The Prostate Answer Book. New York: Warner Books, 1993.
Bostwick, David G, MacLennan, Gregory T, Larson, Thayne R. The American Cancer Society. Prostate Cancer: What Every Man—and His Family—Needs to Know. New York: Villard Books, 1996.

Garnick, Marc B. The Patient's Guide to Prostate Cancer. New York: Penguin Books, 1996.

Gelbard, Martin. Solving Prostate Problems. New York: Fireside, 1995.

Gomellaa, Leonard G, Fried, John J. Recovering From Prostate Cancer: A Doctor's Guide for Patients and Their Loved Ones. New York: Harper Paperbacks, 1993.

Kaltenbach, Don, Richards, Tim. Prostate Cancer: A Survivor's Guide. New Port Richey, Fla.: Seneca House Press, 1995 (S)

Korda, Michael. Man to Man: Surviving Prostate Cancer. New York: Random House, 1996. (S)

Lewis, James Jr. How I Survived Prostate Cancer and So Can You. Westbury, N.Y. (S)

Lifelines: A Guide to Life With Prostate Cancer (videotape). Deerfield, Ill.: TAP Pharmaceuticals.

Marks, Sheldon. Prostate Cancer: A Family Guide to Diagnosis, Treatment, and Survival. Tucson, Ariz.: Fisher Books, 1995.

Martin, William H. My Prostate and Me. New York: Cadell & Davies, 1994. (S)

McDougal, W Scott, Skerrett, PJ. Prostate Disease. New York: Times Books, 1996.

Meyer, Sylvan, Nash, Seymour C. Prostate Cancer: Making Survival Decisions. Chicago: The University of Chicago Press, 1994.

Morganstern, Steven, Abrahams, Alan. The Prostate Source Book: Everything You Need to Know. Los Angeles: Lowell House, 1993.

Payne, James E. Me Too: A Doctor Survives Prostate Cancer. Waco, Tex.: WRS Publishing, 1995. (S)

Phillips, Robert H. Coping With Prostate Cancer. Garden City Park, N.Y.: Avery Publishing Group, 1994.

Rous, Stephen N. The Prostate Book: Sound Advice on Symptoms and Treatment. New York, WW Norton, 1992.

Wainrib, Barbara Rubin, Haber, Sandra, McGuire, Jack. Prostate Cancer: A Guide for Women and the Men They Love. New York: Dell Publishing, 1996.

Walsh, Patrick C, Worthing, Janet Farrar. The Prostate: A Guide for Men and the Women Who Love Them. Baltimore: The Johns Hopkins Press, 1995.

Index

Authors

Allen E. Salowe is a Senior Fellow at the Florida Institute of Education, State University System (SUS), Jacksonville, Florida; a Senior Fellow at the Florida Center for Electronic Communications (SUS), Florida Atlantic University, Ft. Lauderdale, Florida; and an Adjunct Professor at Webster University, Jacksonville, Florida. He is a member of the American Institute of Certified Planners (AICP); and former vice president of ITT Community Development Corporation, Palm Coast, Florida.

Michael J. Wehle, M.D., is a consultant in Urology at the Mayo Clinic Jacksonville, Jacksonville, Florida; and former Associate Clinical Professor at the University of California–San Diego School of Medicine, San Diego, California.

Contributors

Harrison A. Fertig, M.D., F.A.C.C. (retired), is former Chief of Cardiology, Muhlenberg Regional Medical Center, Plainfield, New Jersey; and former Clinical Professor of Medicine, University of Medicine and Dentistry of New Jersey, Robert Wood Johnson School of Medicine, New Brunswick, New Jersey.

Leon M. Lessinger, Ed.D., is an Eminent Scholar in Education Policy and Economic Development and Senior Fellow, Florida Institute of Education, Jacksonville, Florida; former Clinical Professor of Medicine, UCLA Medical Center, Los Angeles, California; former Associate U.S. Commissioner of Education; and former Dean of College of Education, University of South Carolina, Columbia, South Carolina.

M. Brooke Moran is the Director of Patient Advocacy and Government Affairs for the American Foundation for Urologic Diseases (A.F.U.D.), Baltimore, Maryland; editor of the Prostate Cancer Research Directory; and founding trustee of the National Prostate Cancer Coalition (NPCC).

Henry A. Porterfield is Chairman and CEO of US TOO! International, Inc., Hinsdale, Illinois, a not-for-profit resource organization serving men with prostate cancer and prostate disease.

Ordering Information

Additional copies of *Prostate Cancer: Overcoming Denial With Action—A Guide to Screening, Treatment, and Healing* or any of QMP's consumer health books listed below may be purchased from most booksellers, via e-mail, from our home page on the Internet at http://www.qmp.com, by fax, or by mailing the following order form. Substantial discounts on orders of 10 or more books are also available. For information, call QMP's Special Sales Division toll-free at 1-800-348-7808.

Book Title	Price Each	No. Copies	Total Price
Prostate Cancer: Overcoming Denial With Action—A Guide to Screening, Treatment, and Healing ISBN: 1-57626-023-2	$15.00	_____	_____
The Patient's Little Instruction Book ISBN: 1-57626-022-4	$10.00	_____	_____
A Woman's Decision: Breast Care, Treatment & Reconstruction, 2nd ed. ISBN: 1-942219-04-X	$18.50	_____	_____
What Women Need To Know About Breast Self-Examination ISBN: 1-942219-99-6	$ 1.95	_____	_____
What Women Want To Know About Breast Implants ISBN: 1-942219-61-9	$ 6.00	_____	_____
Understanding Managed Health Care: A Guide for Seniors on Medicare ISBN: 1-57626-021-6	$ 6.50	_____	_____

POSTAGE & HANDLING:
$3.00 for first book; $2.00 for each additional book

Postage & Handling   _____

Amount Enclosed   _____

METHOD OF PAYMENT: ❏ Check enclosed
❏ Charge my credit card: ❏ MC   ❏ VISA   ❏ AMEX
\# _____ Exp. date _____
Signature _____

SHIP ORDER TO:
Name _____
Address _____
City/State/Zip _____

Mail this form with payment to: Quality Medical Publishing, Inc.
11970 Borman Drive, Suite 222, St. Louis, MO 63146

Or: Phone: 1-800-348-7808 • Fax: 1-314-878-9937 • e-mail: qmp@qmp.com

WITHDRAWN